Using Patient Reported Outcomes to Improve Health Care

D1333665

Using Patient Reported Outcomes to Improve Health Care

John Appleby

Nancy Devlin

David Parkin

WILEY Blackwell

This edition first published 2016 © 2016 by John Wiley & Sons Ltd

Registered office: John Wiley & Sons, Ltd, The Atrium, Southern Gate, Chichester, West Sussex, PO19 8SQ, UK

Editorial offices: 9600 Garsington Road, Oxford, OX4 2DQ, UK

The Atrium, Southern Gate, Chichester, West Sussex, PO19 8SQ, UK

111 River Street, Hoboken, NJ 07030–5774, USA

For details of our global editorial offices, for customer services and for information about how to apply for permission to reuse the copyright material in this book please see our website at www.wiley.com/wiley-blackwell

Library of Congress Cataloging-in-Publication Data

Appleby, John, 1958- , author.
  Using patient reported outcomes to improve health care / John Appleby, Nancy Devlin, David Parkin.
      p. ; cm.
  Includes bibliographical references and index.
  ISBN 978-1-118-94860-6 (cloth)
  I. Devlin, N. J. (Nancy J.), author. II. Parkin, David W., author. III. Title.
  [DNLM: 1. Patient Outcome Assessment. 2. Data Collection. 3. Delivery of Health Care–organization & administration.
  4. Quality Improvement. W 84.41]
  R853.087
  362.1072'7–dc23

2015029809

A catalogue record for this book is available from the British Library.

Wiley also publishes its books in a variety of electronic formats. Some content that appears in print may not be available in electronic books.

ISBNs

paperback:	978-111-894860-6
ePDF:	978-111-894859-0
epub:	978-111-894858-3

Cover image: GettyImages-185008611/Health Questionaire/Vishwanath Bhat
Gettyimages-493216259/Surgeons performing surgery in operation theatre/Morsa Images

Set in 9/11 and Frutiger LT Std by Aptara Inc., New Delhi, India
Printed and bound in Malaysia by Vivar Printing Sdn Bhd

1 2016

Contents

Foreword

Sir Bruce Keogh
National Medical Director
NHS England
London

The cartoonist's caricature depicted by the caption, 'the operation was a success, but the patient died', defines the problem that patient reported outcome measures aspire to solve – namely a deeper understanding of the relationship between technical and perceived outcomes for a clinical intervention. Patients and surgeons enter into a deal to try and solve a patient's particular problem but expectations are sometimes different. Patient reported outcome measures offer the prospect of employing different and sophisticated tools for measuring and defining a spectrum of success from a patient standpoint which will inevitably facilitate greater patient participation in the decision-making process. This is in keeping with a wider secular trend to give individuals more control over different aspects of their lives, transactions and health. When linked to pre-operative symptoms, procedural data and other clinical outcome measures they offer addition objective measures that could provide a valuable tool for refining and improving surgical interventions and defining their relative value.

The history of surgical outcome measurement has been driven by a desire to improve patient outcomes and hindered by fears of how comparative outcomes may be used. Unravelling the relative utility of different PROMs to patients, clinicians or institutions will require rigorous analysis. This book does just that. It summarises the current state of knowledge, exposes the gaps, explores our experience in the English National Health Service and presents opportunities for future endeavour.

Foreword

An international perspective

Professor Kalipso Chalkidou
Director, NICE International
London

In December 2012 the General Assembly of the United Nations adopted a resolution on universal health care, urging member states to establish health care systems that offer their people access to care they need whilst protecting them from impoverishment due to catastrophic spending. Critics of this global movement claim it is unaffordable – or that what could be afforded by most countries is likely to be of too poor a quality. This is not surprising given that groups such as the World Bank and the World Health Organization have traditionally focused on mechanisms for financing for universal health care. Quality, as linked to costs and affordability in the context of expanding access to needed care, has largely been omitted from the discussion.

Patient reported outcomes (PROs) can change all this. A pragmatic measure of quality, they link effectiveness with efficiency of care, focusing on: '...the impact that a person's state of health has on his or her overall life.' And in doing so is perhaps one of the most powerful tools for supporting nations' efforts to attain and sustain universal health care.

Quality can make or break universal health care. In developing countries, weak clinical governance structures, limited or no professional (self)-regulation, badly behaving pharma and devices industries and confused and distortionary payment systems fuel supply-induced demand, leading to overuse, waste, unsatisfactory patient experiences and bad outcomes.

Doctors in China and India will tell you their patients are 'forcing' them to prescribe IV antibiotics whatever the underlying condition. In Vietnam, providers claim their clients are upset if not offered an MRI scan when admitted to hospital; again, with the underlying condition being of little relevance to the treatment offered. And in many Latin American countries such as Colombia and Costa Rica, patients and their families take public payers to court for not offering them the latest cancer drug, even when such drugs remain unlicensed in the United States or Europe or of poor value for money – even for richer nations.

Patient reported outcomes can challenge all this. They can empower patients in making choices about their treatment based on systematically captured experiences of other patients. They can strengthen third party payers in their attempts to measure and reward performance. They can boost policy makers' efforts in making sense of and tackling unwarranted variation within and across countries. They can help expose links between deprivation and health outcomes and help better target resources. Most interesting for the work NICE International is doing around the world, PROs can bring value for money estimations closer to the realities of front-line medicine as this is practiced in each country's and region's setting instead of relying largely on US-run regulatory trials, fairly unrepresentative of real world comparative effectiveness especially in poorer settings.

Foreword

With the English NHS showing the way, countries around the world are becoming increasingly interested in PROs. On a recent visit to China, physicians in the cardiovascular ward at the brand new Huangdao district hospital, near the North-Eastern port city of Qing Dao, showed me hundreds of completed PRO questionnaires collected as part of an evaluation of a project for improving stroke prevention and management. The Clinical Pathways project, run together with NICE and the Chinese Ministry of Health and supported by the Department for International Development (DFID), is now being rolled out across 500 counties, all encouraged to collect and report on PROs.

Emerging economies, investing more of their own money in health care and faced with growing expectations by their citizens living in increasingly unequal societies, are looking for means of informing their health care policies and coverage decisions. The Vice-Premier of Vietnam has committed his government to improving the quality of health care as a key priority for his government. South Africa, committed to achieving universal health care in the coming decade, last year set up the Office of Healthcare Standards and Compliance, to measure and reward quality. In Thailand – a universal health care success story and a model for developing countries – the National Health Security Office decides on scaling up new services such as dialysis and transplantation based on health technology assessments using results from real world pilots and real world outcomes.

While middle income economies are moving towards measuring quality in the journey to universal health care, poorer countries will need financial support. But there are already huge sums spent through global health and health care aid funds, which could play an increasing role. The Global Fund to Fight AIDS, Tuberculosis and Malaria and the GAVI – the vaccines alliance – and both supported by DFID, could include PROs in their measurements, in part as a means of increasing accountability between them and their funders, but most importantly, between service users in the countries they work in, and providers of aid money. Equally, PROs can serve as a powerful tool for the World Bank's multi-million Health Results Innovation Trust Fund, again co-funded by DFID, and set up to support results based financing. What better way to measure (and reward) health results than with data produced by the actual beneficiaries of aid – patients and the public.

In their recent inquiry into DFID, the International Development Committee of the UK's Parliament emphasised the importance of strengthening health systems whilst measuring real impact, beyond the formulaic metrics of disease or technology specific programmes. PROs can be one such measure of health system strengthening, one that promotes transparency, and with it, strengthens health systems' governance and accountability.

In a world where rich and poor countries have a lot more in common than some may think, lessons and experience from the application of PROs in the NHS can help shape global policy and accelerate the move towards universal health care.

Acknowledgements

The authors are grateful to all our colleagues, from a wide range of institutions around the world, who shared our enthusiasm about the use of health outcomes in health care systems, and kindly agreed to contribute material for this book. We are also grateful to the King's Fund and the Office of Health Economics for allowing us to update and further develop an initial version of this book which was published jointly by those two institutions in 2010.

In particular, we would like to thank Sir Bruce Keogh and Professor Kalipso Chalkidou for their forewords to this book, and to Jo Partington, Jeffrey Johnson, Christopher Smith, Carolyn De Coster, Tim Hughes, Ray Naden, Alison Barber, Evalill Nilsson, Kristina Burström, Andrew Vallance-Owen, Jiaying Chen and Yaling Yang for their contributions.

John Appleby
Nancy Devlin
David Parkin
London 2015

Acknowledgements

CHAPTER 1

Introduction

The ultimate measure by which to judge the quality of a medical effort is whether it helps patients (and their families) as they see it. Anything done in health care that does not help a patient or family is, by definition, waste, whether or not the professions and their associations traditionally hallow it. (Berwick, 1997: Reproduced with permission of BMJ Publishing Group Ltd.)

The goal of most health care is to improve patients' health and there is a strong argument that patients themselves are the people best placed to judge how their state of health affects them. There is a growing recognition throughout the world's health care systems that the patient's perspective on health and health care is highly relevant to – and indeed, needs to be at the heart of – efforts to improve the quality and effectiveness of health care.

Information provided by patients about their health does not replace clinical measures of health and illness. But it can provide valuable, complementary information about how health problems and the effects of health care interventions are experienced by patients. These data, carefully collected and appropriately analysed, can provide crucial insights about the patients view on health, and the quality of health care, that would otherwise be missed.

There has been a considerable investment of resources by academics and clinicians, spanning the last three decades, to develop systematic, robust and valid ways of collecting self-reported health data from patients. These efforts have resulted in the availability of Patient Reported Outcomes questionnaires (PROs).

In broad terms, PROs comprise a series of structured questions that ask patients about their health from their point of view. There are now literally thousands of questionnaires available for measuring patient reported outcomes. Carefully collected PRO data from patients are likely to become a key part of how all health care is funded, provided and managed in the future.

PRO questionnaires are already very widely used in clinical trials and observational studies, alongside clinical end-points, and those data are widely recognised as providing a vital part of the evidence required in decisions to approve and make pricing and reimbursement decisions about new health care technologies. Well-established Health Technology Appraisal (HTA) bodies, charged with a responsibility to judge the effectiveness and value for money of new treatments, such as the UK's National Institute for Health and Care Excellence (NICE), require PRO evidence to be submitted as part of their deliberations (NICE, 2013). In that context, PRO data are often used to estimate the Quality Adjusted Life Years (QALYs)[1] gained by patients receiving new therapies.

---

[1] QALYs are a generic measure of length and quality of life – capturing the two main outcomes/goals of health care: to prolong life and improve its quality.

Using Patient Reported Outcomes to Improve Health Care,
First Edition. John Appleby, Nancy Devlin and David Parkin.
© 2016 John Wiley & Sons, Ltd. Published 2016 by John Wiley & Sons, Ltd.

PROs have also long been included in population health surveys, as a means of measuring population health and morbidity (see Szende *et al.*, 2014) The population norms provided by such surveys help policy makers understand what 'normal' health means, from the perspective of people of various socio-demographic backgrounds, in local communities. That provides a baseline for understanding the burden of disease from illnesses, and is used to inform priorities for resource allocation decisions.

However, the use of PROs, until very recently, tended to be limited to one-off studies of general or patient populations. The use of PROs in the real world context of health care delivery settings is relatively new.

The possibility of routinely collecting and using these data alongside the delivery of care was first recognised by the private sector in the UK. Bupa, the UK's biggest private health insurer and (at that time) owner of a network of private hospital, asked its patients to complete PRO questionnaires before and after a number of elective surgical procedures. The data were used to monitor and benchmark the quality of care by its surgical teams. The routine use of patient reported outcomes was introduced into the English National Health Service (NHS) in 2009. Known as the PROMs (Patient Reported Outcome Measures) programme, it was a landmark development in the use of PROs across an entire whole health care system. The move has attracted considerable interest elsewhere, and other health care systems are now following suit.

The economic context

Health care accounts for a substantial and growing proportion of both overall economic activity and government spending in developed economies. In 2012, for example, total (public and private) spending on health care accounted for 9.3% of the aggregate GDP for the 34 countries comprising the OECD. In the US, around one dollar in six of the entire economy is now devoted to health care. In the Netherlands, around one Euro in eight and in France and Germany, one Euro in ten. Since the 1960s, most OECD countries have seen the proportion of GDP devoted to health care more or less double. Health care also absorbs a significant proportion of government spending – especially in countries such as the UK that have predominantly tax-funded health care systems and where the NHS accounts for nearly a fifth of all government.

But what is *produced* from health care spending? What *value* does expenditure on health services generate for patients and for economies? While most other sectors of the economy generate outputs that can readily be measured and valued – quantities of goods and services, and the prices at which they are bought and sold – in contrast, health services have traditionally posed considerable challenges for the measurement of output and productivity (Office of Health Economics, 2008). For example, following the historically unprecedented increases in real spending on the NHS in the years following 2000, commentators reasonably asked: where did the money go? What was achieved by the massive increase in spending?

In stark contrast, the current economic environment in which the English NHS and other health care systems operate has changed dramatically as a result of the financial crisis and recession of 2008–2009 (Appleby *et al.*, 2014). Since that time, the NHS has had to adjust to zero or small real increases in spending (Appleby *et al.*, 2009a), against a backdrop of constantly rising demand. Notwithstanding the changed economic context, the questions remain essentially the same:

- Can we be sure that public spending on health care is justified by the outputs that it produces?
- Are scarce public sector resources being used in a way that maximises their value to patients and society?

- How do different sorts of health care services, that we could spend our money on, compare in terms of their effectiveness and value for money in improving patient health?
- How do different providers of health care compare in terms of their performance in improving patient health?

Special issues with measuring and valuing health

Assessing the output and productivity of health care poses special problems. Health care services or products themselves are easy to record and count: the number of hospital admissions, doctors' visits, surgical procedures undertaken, tooth cavities filled, prescriptions issued, and so on. But these cannot simply be added up to give an indication of what is produced overall. More importantly, they are *intermediate* outputs. Most health services are not valued in their own right, but rather because of the effects they have on something much more fundamental: health. Health is the true final output of health care.

Yet efforts to measure the health produced by health care systems such as the English NHS have been fairly rudimentary. Traditional measures have tended to focus on the prevalence of adverse outcomes, such as post-surgical mortality, hospital-acquired infections and readmission rates. It is, of course, important to know about these bad things, and they do need to be minimised. But such incidents are also relatively rare and shed little light on the great majority of health service interventions for most patients.

As a basis for assessing the value of the vast resources devoted to health care in the world's health care systems, however, these measures are hopelessly inadequate.

The purpose of a health care system is not just to minimise the harm caused by its activity, but also (and arguably, principally) to produce health and social benefits for patients and society. Despite a century of developments in medical technology, and vast improvements in the ability of medical science to prevent, diagnose and treat disease and ill health, attempts to measure the outputs of health care in terms of their impact on patients' health have barely progressed beyond Florence Nightingale's time. More than 100 years ago, she suggested a simple three-point health-related outcome measure for her patients: relieved; unrelieved; and dead (Appleby and Devlin, 2004).

Clinicians have, of course developed measures to guide and inform their clinical practice. These provide important and relevant information about the impact of health care interventions on clinically defined variables, but, while useful, they typically fail to inform wider questions crucial to measuring the *overall* output and quality of health care services.

Moreover, the many different clinical indicators used in medical practice do not always distinguish the aspects of health that patients consider important, or their relative value to patients. The observation that 'the operation was a success, but the patient died' might be an example of the dark humour of the medical profession, but it is nonetheless indicative of the gap that can exist between the views of clinicians and patients on what matters in health care.

Furthermore, the many different clinical measures used make it hard to compare health impacts across specialties. It is therefore difficult to draw any conclusions about the overall effects of spending and service delivery across different disease areas, or their ultimate effects on health outcomes. Nor is it possible to identify how those outcomes could be improved by different allocations of resources between services and patients.

In addition, although patient-reported experience measures (sometimes referred to as PREMs) can provide useful indications of patients' perspectives and views about the care they have received, by their nature these reflect experience of the *process* rather than the *outcome* of care. As the final report of the NHS Next Stage Review observes, '…just as important is the effectiveness of care from the patient's own perspective, which will be measured through patient reported outcomes measures…' (Department of Health, 2008).

It is clear that a fundamental rethink about what 'outputs' and 'outcomes' mean in health care is long overdue.

A fundamental shift in focus

Against this backdrop, there has been a marked shift internationally in thinking about what health is and how it is measured. Traditional clinical ways of measuring health and the effects of treatment are increasingly accompanied by, or indeed replaced by, PROs.

This shift in focus is most evident in the appraisal of new health care technologies, where products and practices are subject to rigorous evaluation. The United States' Food and Drug Administration (FDA), which has recently recommended the inclusion of PROs in US clinical trials (Food and Drug Administration, 2006), notes: 'The use of PRO instruments is part of a general movement toward the idea that the patient, properly queried, is the best source of information about how he or she feels' (Bren, 2006).

In parts of the English NHS, most notably in the work done by the NICE in appraising the effectiveness and cost effectiveness of new health care technologies, the use of PRO data is already commonplace. Indeed, pharmaceutical companies are required to submit evidence on PROs to support NICE's Health Technology Appraisal (HTA) process (NICE, 2013). Similar HTA processes, utilising PRO data, are also in place in a range of other countries including Canada, Sweden, Australia and New Zealand, and with interest in the development of HTA in many of the large, emerging economies shifting toward collectively funded health care systems, such as China and Brazil.

Over the course of several decades, clinical, health services and social sciences research-ers have produced literally thousands of validated instruments that facilitate the consistent, reliable measurement of patient-reported health. Patients' perspectives on their health out-comes can now be measured in most clinical areas.

Routine measurement of PROs: a step forward in the NHS

An important development in this area took place in the English NHS in England in April 2009. The Department of Health introduced a requirement for the routine measurement of patient-reported health outcomes for all NHS patients in England before and after receiving surgery, via its Patient Reported Outcome Measures (PROMs) programme (Department of Health, 2007, 2008a). Box 1.2 provides some key facts about the NHS PROMs programme, and activities underway for its extension. Appendix 1 shows the PROM questionnaire that is currently completed by patients after undergoing varicose vein surgery.

Box 1.2 Key facts about the implementation of the PROMs programme in the NHS in England

Jo Partington[2]

In 2009 the routine collection of PROs from patients, both before and after NHS-funded surgery, was introduced by the English Department of Health for four elective procedures:

- hip replacement
- knee replacement

- varicose veins
- hernia

Those data are now being used in a wide range of ways including:

- To measure the outcomes of the health care system under the Government's 'Outcomes Framework'
- To performance-manage organisations providing NHS treatment, as well as incentivising good outcomes by including patient outcomes in payment mechanisms (e.g. the Hip/Knee Best Practice Tariff from April 2014).
- Regulatory bodies, such as Care Quality Commission, use PROMs programme data in their intelligence monitoring.
- Patients and their GPs can use PROMs data, published on the health and Social Care Information Centre website, to inform their choice of providers at the point of referral.

Following restructuring of the health care system, responsibility for the PROMs programme passed from the Department of Health to NHS England.

An important development has been the collection of PRO data in the GP patient survey (GPPS). Since 2011–2012, the generic PRO used in the PROMs programme, the EQ-5D, has also been included in the GPPS. Data are collected from around 900 000 patients each year, half of whom have long term conditions. The data are being used to produce new insights into questions about primary care, and the effects of multimorbidities on patient health.

Pilot studies have been undertaken to explore the possibility of extending PROMs over a wider range of conditions and treatments in the NHS, including:

- mental health, for example anxiety and depression
- cancer care
- six long-term conditions: asthma, COPD, diabetes, epilepsy, heart failure, stroke
- cancers of the breast, prostate, bowel, Non-Hodgkin's Lymphoma.

NHS England NHS England is involved in a number of pilots being analysed/evaluated in the following areas:

- revascularisation;
- cancers of the bladder, womb, cervix or ovary.

In addition, pilots are currently being developed for PROMs in

- Musculoskeletal,
- Renal replacement,
- Major trauma,
- Dementia.

In addition, work is underway for the inclusion of PROMs data collection in National Clinical Audits. In each case, the approach to potentially the extending the PROMs programme comprises the following careful process:

- identifying the appropriate PROM instruments
- piloting their use and reviewing their potential to be rolled out across the NHS
- implementing data collection and related procedures
- evaluating the programme.

Progression depends on there being sufficient evidence at each stage to support the use of PROMs. To date mandated PROMs are limited to the initial four elective procedures.

[2] Patient Reported Outcome Measures Insight Account Manager, NHS England.

The requirement to collect PRO data introduced applied to just four surgical procedures — hernia repair, hip and knee replacement and varicose veins. Those four procedures cost the NHS in England around £800 million per year. Since its introduction, around quarter of a million patients have been invited each year be to complete questionnaires both before and after surgery. All NHS providers are currently collecting these data. A very good response rate has been achieved, for example 80% in hip replacement patients. The annual cost of the current PROMs programme is estimated to represent less than 0.5% of expenditure on the relevant interventions.

The NHS PROMs programme is an extraordinary achievement, both in terms of the proven logistics of large scale data collection, and in terms of its ambition in using routinely collected health outcomes data to drive health care decision making.

However, progress in further developing the NHS PROMs programme since that date has been slow. Pilot work is under way to explore the feasibility of and case for extending routine measurement to a range of chronic conditions, including diabetes, asthma, stroke, chronic obstructive pulmonary disease (COPD) and others (see Box 1.2). Contingent on there being positive evidence to support their use, the routine collection of PRO data could be introduced across a wide range of NHS services.

PRO data are used across a range of applications, including measuring and managing hospitals in their efforts to improve patient health. Indicators of hospital performance, based on PROs, are to be included in the information provided to patients being referred for elective surgery, to assist them in choosing the hospital at which they will receive treatment.

This reflects a key theme of various changes in the NHS since the turn of the century, namely to improve the responsiveness of the NHS to patients' views, preferences and choices. Research has indicated that patients regard the relative performance of providers in improving their health as highly important in choosing where to receive surgery (Burge *et al.*, 2006), yet to date it has been the aspect of performance about which least information existed.

The PROMs initiative is a truly remarkable development for the NHS — and a first internationally: the NHS will be the first health care system in the world to measure what it produces in terms of *health*, rather than in terms of the production of *health care*. The intention is that, in addition to clinical measures of outcome, PROs will enable patient perspectives to be taken into account in key aspects of the NHS, including:

- informing the choices patients make with regard to their treatment and its providers
- measuring and benchmarking the performance of health care providers
- linking the payment received by providers to their performance in improving patient health
- understanding and managing referral from primary to secondary care
- facilitating cooperation between clinicians and managers in the delivery of care
- enabling health care professionals to monitor and improve health care practices
- regulating for safety and quality in health care services.

As the potential scope of the PROMs programme in the NHS could extend beyond elective surgery, these data will offer a powerful new means of managing the performance of the NHS.

Getting the most out of patient reported outcomes

The aim of this book is to provoke and encourage thinking about the wide range of ways in which PRO data, routinely collected in the context of health service delivery, can be used to inform decisions.

- What opportunities do these data present?
- What are the limitations of PROs and what are the possible pitfalls in the use and over-interpretation of data produced from them?
- What work needs to be done in order to get the most out of PRO data?
- What have been the experiences of the English NHS with its PROs programme and what can be learned from that by other health care systems?

In the next chapter, we provide an overview and explanation of PRO instruments. Then in Chapter 3 we look first at how PRO data might be used by patients in choosing both *where* to receive treatment, and also *what* treatment is best for them; and then we consider other ways in which the data now being collected can be used to transform decision making in the NHS (and, by extension, in any health care system anywhere in the world).

We then consider, in Chapter 4, how clinicians might use these data. Drawing on the experience of the Canadian and New Zealand health care systems, we consider whether there is scope for using PRO data to guide referral practices, to ensure that the people who receive health care are those that will benefit from it the most.

Following on from this, Chapter 5 discusses how providers can use the data to benchmark and improve clinical performance within their own organisations, drawing on the example of Bupa.

In Chapter 6, we look at how PROs might be used by those who commission health care on behalf of patients to assess value for money and purchase health care services that maximise improvement in the health of the communities they serve. We also consider the possibility of commissioners directly linking provider reimbursement to PROs performance.

Chapter 7 shows how measuring improvements in patient health can address high-level questions about productivity and performance in the NHS.

We conclude by asking the question 'Where next for PROs?' Routine use of PROs has the potential to put the views and values of patients squarely at the heart of health care systems management and clinical thinking about the provision of health care services. Our aim is to help ensure that these benefits are realised and that the NHS and other health care systems maximise the benefit to patients that collecting these data makes possible.

References

Appleby J, Crawford R, Emmerson C (2009a) *How Cold Will It Be? Prospects for NHS Funding 2011–17*. London: King's Fund/Institute for Fiscal Studies. Available at: www.kingsfund.org.uk/sites/files/kf/How-Cold-Will-It-Be-Prospects-NHS-funding-2011-2017-John-Appleby-Roweena_Crawford-Carl-Emmerson-The-Kings-Fund-July-2009.pdf (accessed on 1 July 2015).

Appleby J, Devlin N (2004) *Measuring Success in the NHS. Using Patient-Assessed Health Outcomes to Manage the Performance of Health Care Providers*. London: King's Fund/Dr Foster.

Appleby J, Helderman J-K, Gregory S (2014) The global financial crisis, health and health care *Health Economics, Policy and Law*, vol 10, pp 1–6 (available at http://journals.cambridge.org/action/displayFulltext?type=1&fid=9454394&jid=HEP&volumeId=10&issueId=01&aid=9454370&bodyId=&membershipNumber=&societyETOCSession=, accessed 15 June, 2015).

Berwick DM (1997) Medical associations: guilds or leaders. *British Medical Journal*, vol 314, no 7094, pp 1564–1565.

Bren L (2006) The importance of patient reported outcomes…It's all about the patients. FDA Consumer, November–December issue. Silver Spring, MD: Food and Drug Administration. Available at: http://permanent.access.gpo.gov/lps1609/www.fda.gov/fdac/features/2006/606_patients.html (accessed on 1 July 2015).

Burge, P, Devlin, N, Appleby J, Gallo F, Nason E, Ling T (2006) Understanding Patients' Choices at the Point of Referral. *Technical report TR359-DOH*. Cambridge: RAND Europe. Available at: www .rand.org/pubs/technical_reports/TR359/ (accessed on 15 June, 2015).

Department of Health (2007) *Guidance of the Routine Collection of Patient Reported Outcome Measures (PROMs)*. London: Department of Health.

Department of Health (2008a) *Guidance on the Routine Collection of Patient Reported Outcome Measures (PROMs)*. For the NHS in England 2009/10. London: Department of Health. Available at: http://webarchive.nationalarchives.gov.uk/20130107105354/www.dh.gov.uk/en/ Publicationsandstatistics/Publications/PublicationsPolicyAndGuidance/DH_091443 (accessed on 1 July 2015).

Food and Drug Administration (2006) *Guidance for Industry: Patient-reported outcome measures: use in medical product development to support labeling claims: draft guidance*. Rockville, MD: US Department of Health and Human Services Food and Drug Administration. Available at: www.ncbi.nlm.nih.gov/pmc/articles/PMC1629006/ (accessed on 1 July 2015).

National Institute for Health and Care Excellence (NICE) (2013) *Guide to the Methods of Technology Appraisal 2013*. Available at: http://publications.nice.org.uk/pmg9 (accessed 15 June, 2015).

Office of Health Economics (2008) *Report of the Office of Health Economics Commission on NHS Outcomes, Performance and Productivity*. London: Office of Health Economics.

Szende A, Janssen, B, Cabases, J (eds) (2014) *Measuring self-reported population health: Self-Reported Population Health: An International Perspective based on EQ-5D*. Dordrecht, The Netherlands: Springer.

CHAPTER 2

A primer on patient reported outcomes

What are PROs?

A patient-reported outcome (PRO) questionnaire is a series of questions that patients are asked in order to gauge their views on their own health. The name is fairly self-explanatory: PROs are completed by *patients* themselves. The purpose of PROs is to get patients' own assessments of their *health* and *health-related quality of life*. PRO questionnaires do not ask about patients' satisfaction with or experience of health care services, or seek their opinions about how successful their treatment was. In their use in the English NHS, PROs are often referred to as PROMs - Patient Reported Outcome Measures.

In the various uses of PROs that are the focus of this book, it is *patients* who answer the questions, but these same questions are often included in surveys designed to measure health among the general population, such as the annual Health Survey for England commissioned by the English Department of Health. In those contexts, the 'P' in PROs could just as easily stand for 'person' rather than 'patient'. The main thing about a PRO is that health is assessed by the person experiencing it, not by a doctor or anyone else.

The questions can be asked by paper and pencil questionnaires, interviews, or, increasingly commonly, by electronic means, for example a computer or handheld electronic device.

Measuring health using patient questionnaires is not new, and the label 'Patient Reported Outcomes' is to a great extent simply a re-labelling of the largest element of a clinical and academic activity called Health Status Measurement (Bowling, 2001; 2004). There are literally thousands of different PRO questionnaires or instruments, differing in terms of the wording and nature of the questions asked, the number of questions asked, and how the answers are scored or summed up. The quality of these instruments, in terms of their reliability and validity, can vary considerably. The particular instruments currently being used in the NHS PROMs programme were chosen by the Department of Health after careful consideration and testing in pilot studies (Browne *et al.*, 2007).

The various PRO instruments (sets of questions) available fall into a number of distinct types. The most important differences/types are summarised in Table 2.1 and are explained in the following.

Using Patient Reported Outcomes to Improve Health Care,
First Edition. John Appleby, Nancy Devlin and David Parkin.

Table 2.1 A taxonomy of different types of PROs, with examples

How is health summarised?	How is health described?	
	Generic	Condition-specific
Scores	The most widely used instrument of this sort is the SF-36 (Ware and Sherbourne, 1992). It comprises 36 questions. The patient's health is then summarised by a mental health component score and a physical health component score. There is no overall score.	There are literally thousands of questionnaires designed for specific conditions – from respiratory conditions to depression.
Value	The most widely used instrument of this sort in the United Kingdom and Europe is the EQ-5D (Brooks, 1996). Patients answer five questions, each concerning a different dimension of their health. They also provide an overall assessment of their health, on visual analogue scale (VAS), ranging from 0 (worst possible health) to 100 (best possible health). The patient's health, as he or she describes it on the five dimensions, can also be given a value that represents society's views about that state. These values are available in EQ-5D value sets, which are based on the views and preferences of the general public, asked to imagine living in EQ-5D health states. NICE, for example, uses these data in estimating quality adjusted life year (QALY) gains.	None of the condition-specific measures claims to capture patients' *overall* quality of life, nor the value patients or society place on that. However, some condition specific instruments are accompanied by values used in estimating QALYs, in the same way as for generic PROs.

How do PROs measure health?

Some PROs set out to describe or measure health in a way that is general (or generic), so that the same questions can be used for patients with completely different conditions, and so that health and changes in health can be compared across different patient and population groups. These generic instruments measure health in terms of the effect of any given state of health on the ability to function and enjoy life, which is why they are sometimes referred to as measures of Quality of Life (QoL) or health-related quality of life (HRQOL). The focus is on the *impact* that a person's state of health has on his or her overall life.

Because generic PROs measure health in a general way, they are used in population health surveys, where the objective is to assess and compare the health of communities of people. For example, Szende *et al.* (2014) provide an overview of the use of one such instrument, the EQ-5D, in international studies of population health. Generic PROs are also crucial to decision makers needing to allocate budgets, where it is important to be able to compare health gain from treatments for one set of patients, with health gain from other treatments, for other patients.

Other sorts of instruments measure patient reported health in a way that is specific to a particular disease, set of conditions or part of the body. In Table 2.1 these are called condition-specific measures, although some are more accurately described as disease-specific measures. The questions in these instruments measure the severity of a particular condition or some specific aspect of health, as viewed by the patient. The questions focus on the particular sorts of limitations or problems that people can experience as a result of a very specific *condition* (e.g. the International Restless Leg Syndrome Study Group rating scale (IRLS; Walters *et al.*, 2003), or ask questions relevant to a wider set of conditions that affect a *body part* (e.g. the Oxford Knee Score; Dawson *et al.*, 1996), or might focus on a particular type of functioning (e.g. the VF-14 measures visual functioning; Steinberg *et al.*, 1994). An important recent addition to the set of condition specific PROs has been the US-based initiative, PROMIS (Patient Reported Outcomes Measurement Information System). PROMIS provides a system of carefully validated measures of patient reported health status for physical, mental and social well-being. A feature of PROMIS is the availability of banks of question items, combined in various ways to create questionnaires.

Condition-specific instruments are relevant to people who suffer, or are suspected of suffering, from particular health problems. They are not usually used in population health surveys.

Both generic and condition-specific PRO questionnaires have as an aim the ability to compare health status or changes in health over time or between patients, either with the same condition (in the case of condition specific PROs) or more generally (in the case of generic PROs). However, there are a further category of PRO instruments which are more focused on the measurement of individual experience of health. An example of these individualised PROs is the Schedule for the Evaluation of Individual Quality of Life (SEIQOL) (O'Boyle, 1994). The distinguishing feature of individualised PROs is that the domains of health that are measured, and the weights attached to them, are driven by what is important to each individual patient.

In the NHS PROMs programme, the questionnaires that patients are asked to complete shortly before and some months after surgery comprise a disease-specific instrument, a generic instrument, and a series of additional questions about the patient's health and symptoms. The EQ-5D, described in more detail in Box 2.1 and, as Box 2.2 details, adopted as the main generic health measure in Alberta, Canada, is used as the generic instrument for each surgical procedure in the English NHS PROMs programme.

For condition-specific measures, the hip and knee replacement questionnaires include the Oxford Knee Score and the Oxford Hip Score (Dawson *et al.*, 1996), respectively, and the Aberdeen Varicose Vein Questionnaire (Garratt *et al.*, 1993) is used for varicose vein repair – there are no such measures for hernia repair.

Box 2.1 The EQ-5D

The EQ-5D (so named because it was developed by the EuroQol Group and has five dimensions) is the generic instrument being used in the NHS PROMs programme in England. It comprises two parts.

In the first part, the patient is asked to describe their health in terms of the levels within each of five dimensions:

- mobility
- self-care
- usual activities
- pain and discomfort
- anxiety and depression.

In the second part of the instrument, patients are asked to provide an overall assessment of their health on a visual analogue scale of 0–100.

The best-known version of the instrument, which has been in widespread use internationally for more than two decades, asks patients to report their health in each dimension by indicating whether they have 'no problems', 'some problems' or 'extreme problems'. This three-level version of the EQ-5D is the one now being used throughout the NHS as part of the PROMs programme (see p. 8 of the questionnaire in Appendix 1).

A newer version of the instrument has recently been published offering five levels within each of the five dimensions, giving patients more options for describing their health (Herdman *et al.*, 2008). Called the EQ-5D-5L, this five-level version is reproduced in Appendix 2.

The five-level version is intended to be more sensitive to changes in health, and includes other improvements (e.g. it no longer uses 'confined to bed' to describe the most severe problems with mobility).

Box 2.2 PROs in Alberta, Canada

Jeffrey Johnson[1], Christopher Smith[2] and Carolyn De Coster[3]

Alberta has established itself as the most active province in Canada to use PROs in clinical and population health settings. Alberta Health's *Health System Outcomes and Measurement Framework* (Alberta Health, 2013) has identified the importance of patient care outcomes, public health outcomes and value for investment. In this light, Alberta Health Services (AHS) has committed to gathering feedback from patients in terms of both their experiences and outcomes.

Since 2010, AHS has captured feedback on patients' experiences using the US-developed Hospital-Consumer Assessment of Healthcare Providers and Systems (H-CAHPS) (Cleary *et al.*, 2012) on a provincial basis. Surveys are done using computer-assisted telephone interviews, currently aiming for 10% of patients within 42 days of discharge from 93 inpatient facilities each year. The latest response rate for the H-CHAPS is approximately 73%. This is an important process, as adult satisfaction with hospital care is one of 16 publicly-reported performance measures for AHS. A similar child inpatient experience survey has also been developed and is being collected for children discharged from the two major children's hospitals in the province. AHS also collects data on patient experience from emergency medical services and for ambulatory cancer care. Data on experience and outcomes for people living in long term care residential sector is also monitored by the Health Quality Council of Alberta (HQCA).

The collection of PROs is less well organised within AHS at present, but a provincial implementation strategy is being developed. A number of groups within the province have implemented PROs programs, with a notable example being the Alberta Bone & Joint Health Institute (ABJHI) for elective total joint arthroplasty. ABJHI, in partnership with AHS and physicians, routinely captures data on the Western Ontario and McMaster Universities Arthritis Index (WOMAC) and the EQ-5D for all patients undergoing hip or knee replacement. These PROMs are used to describe the patient populations in terms of functional status and health-related quality of life, to inform clinics, surgeons and health administrators about patient outcomes and effectiveness of treatment. More recently, ABJHI is using PRO data to develop tools to better predict post-surgery outcomes.

There is also considerable interest in PROs with other provincial organisations. Like AHS, Alberta Health and the HQCA have also identified the EQ-5D as a standard generic instrument for the collection of data on health status of the Alberta population. These organisations are partnering with the School of Public Health at the University of Alberta to establish a novel research unit, which would support end-users of the EQ-5D in the province, while developing an innovative research agenda on the application of the EQ-5D in large-scale health applications. The Alberta EQ-5D Research Unit was established in 2015, with a 5-year commitment by the funding partners. It is based at the University of Alberta, supported by local academics affiliated with the international EuroQol Research Foundation. The Unit will provide leadership, expertise, advice and support for the application of the various EQ-5D instruments, and analysis of EQ-5D and other PRO data collected by various end-user organisations in Alberta, as well as serve as a liaison between Alberta-based end-users and the EuroQol Business Office.

[1] School of Public Health, University of Alberta.
[2] Alberta Bone & Joint Health Institute.
[3] Clinical Analytics & Primary Data Support, Alberta Health Services

It is worth mentioning here developments in user-based measures in social care. Although the main focus of this book is the development and use of measures of health-related quality of life, increasingly the distinction between health and social care services has become blurred – especially in terms of the needs of elderly people and those with long term care conditions. In recognition of this, greater integration between health and social care services and budgets together with a unified approach to commissioning have been advocated (e.g. Barker, 2014). Different countries organise their health and social care services differently; some – at least notionally – run integrated services with single budgets (such as Northern Ireland). Others, such as England have funded and run health and social care services separately – although with a degree of integration at the sharp end of care and some partial efforts in combined funding and commissioning. Overall, the direction of travel from a policy point of view is towards a more integrated approach of one sort or the other. With this in mind, Box 2.3 describes some of the emerging user-based outcome measures in social care.

Box 2.3 Outcome measures for social care?

Just as for health care, there are similar questions concerning the outcomes that social care services and interventions produce, whether competing interventions are cost effective or not and so on. Moreover, there are clear two-way interactions between health and social-care related aspects of quality of life. For these reasons, over the last decade or more there have been various attempts to develop quantifiable quality of life measures related to social care needs that parallel the development in the health care field with generic instruments such as the EQ-5D and the SF-36. Various measures have been developed such as the index of capability ICECAP (Coast et al., 2008). One measure of social-care related quality of life, ASCOT – the adult social care outcomes toolkit (Netten et al., 2012) – is now being used routinely at national level to track changes in quality of life as part of the routine survey of users of adult social care services and has the potential to fulfil a similar role to the EQ-5D in terms of the measurement of outcomes in social care.

The adult social care outcomes toolkit (ASCOT) is a measure similar in many ways to the EQ-5D (and with which it is correlated) but which captures either self-completed or interview or observational information about an individual's social care-related quality of life (Netten *et al.*, 2012).

ASCOT has eight attributes or domains covering: personal cleanliness and comfort, food and drink, control over daily life, personal safety, accommodation cleanliness and comfort, social participation and involvement, occupation and dignity. These can be rated in three levels depending on the version of ASCOT and imply: no needs, low level needs and high needs. A four-level version, the top level is divided to distinguish 'no needs' from the desired situation.

ASCOT also includes a 'hypothetical' question that asks people to rate their quality of life in the absence of services, or their 'expected needs'.

Data collected by ASCOT can be, as with the EQ-5D, analysed in a disaggregated form at the level of the separate domains. However, ASCOT can also be scored to produce a single number by summing domains weighted by the public's relative preference or value for each domain. Weights have been derived from a study of 500 members of the general population.

How is a patient's self-reported health on the various dimensions summarised?

Patients' responses to PRO questionnaires provide detailed information on a variety of aspects of their health and quality of life. However, in order to provide an *overall* assessment of a patient's health, and to make comparisons between, for example, health before and after treatment or between groups of patients, it is necessary to combine the answers the patient has provided on each question into a single score. PRO instruments achieve this in a number of different ways.

One method is to assign a score to each answer, and then add them up to give an overall score. For example, the International Prostate Symptom Score (IPSS) is a condition-specific PRO measure used in urology to measure prostate problems (Barry *et al.*, 1992). (In Chapter 4, there is a detailed discussion of how clinicians use such instruments in their clinical practice, by Professor Mark Emberton, consultant urologist at University College Hospital, London.) The IPSS contains questions such as: 'Over the past month, how many times did you most typically get up to urinate from the time you went to bed until the time you got up in the morning?' There are six possible answers: (a) none; (b) once; (c) twice; (d) three times; (e) four times and (f) five times or more. Each of those answers will be given a score (a) = 0; (b) = 1; (c) = 2; (d) = 3; (e) = 4 and (f) = 5. The overall score is then simply the sum of the scores on each question.

This is the most common procedure used in condition-specific PRO measures. It is often done simply for convenience and without regard for the logic of adding together such diverse elements, but in other cases the scores are tested for their validity – essentially their correlation with other measures of the condition and with expert opinions.

The problem with scoring is that there is an assumption, which is not always explicitly made or tested, that the weight placed both on increasing levels of problems and on each type of problem might not reflect their relative importance to the individual patient answering the questions. It may not be three times as bad to get up in the night to urinate as once and this particular aspect of prostate problems may not have exactly the same importance as other aspects.

Moreover, relying on these overall scores loses some of the descriptive richness of the answers to the individual questions in the PROs, and for some purposes patients' values might not be the most pertinent. For example, in the use of PRO data in Health Technology Appraisal (HTA), where PRO data are used to estimate QALYs for cost effectiveness analysis of new health care technologies, it is often argued that society's values for each health state (i.e. the health state values provided by a representative sample of the general public) should be used, rather than those of patients (NICE, 2013). However, that is not always the case – HTA processes in some countries, such as Sweden, consider patients' values to be more relevant. Ultimately, this question of whose values should be used to summarise PRO data is a normative one.

An alternative is to ask patients themselves to summarise their overall state of health. For example, the second part of the EQ-5D (see Box 2.1), the EQ-VAS, uses a visual, 'thermometer-type' scale to ask patients how they feel overall on a range of 0 (worst possible health) to 100 (best possible health). This might be thought to show how patients value their own health overall and their overall score will reflect both the relative importance they place on the different aspects of their health that are included in the EQ-5D, as well as other dimensions of health that may matter to them. Yan Feng and colleagues have looked in more detail at some of the problems and benefits of this way of asking patients to summarise their health state. They found that this apparently simple way of recording health status may not, in practise, turn out to be as easy as supposed, with only 45% of a sample of 400 completed EQ-VAS measures being completed strictly according to the instructions (Feng et al., 2014). Nevertheless, they argue that the EQ-VAS data provides unambiguous data in the vast majority of cases, and also that the challenges noted could be readily addressed by providing better guidance on collection and coding. Furthermore, it is clear that the EQ-VAS provides important, complementary piece of evidence by telling us about the patients' overall views about their health and quality of life.

Where patients' values are not considered relevant, an alternative is to use values (sometimes also called 'utilities') provided by members of the general public for the health states described by PRO instruments. These values are listed in a *social value set*, obtained via a complex process in which members of the general public are asked to imagine living in the different health states, and then to state their preferences using one of a range of methods designed by economists for that purpose (Morris et al., 2012). Generic PROs for which such value sets (sometimes called *tariffs*) are available include the EQ-5D (Szende et al., 2007), the EQ-5D-5L (e.g. see Devlin et al. 2015 for an EQ-5D-5L value set for England); Health Utilities Index (HUI) (Horsman et al., 2003), Assessment of Quality of Life (AQoL) (Hawthorne et al., 1999) and WHOQOL (WHOQOL Group, 1998). The SF-6D, a shorter version of the SF-36 referred to in Table 2.1 as not having an overall score, has been developed, accompanied by value sets (Kharroubi et al., 2007).

An important thing for users to be aware of is that there is no neutral way of summarising the data which patients provide on PRO questionnaires. *Any* method of combining patients' responses on multiple questions must entail some weight being placed on each question. Even if the *same* weight is placed on each question, that implies a judgement about the relative importance of that kind of health problem to the patient that may or may not reflect the patient's view. Further, the use of value sets to summarise generic PRO data, such as that from the EQ-5D, HUI or SF-6D, introduces an exogenous source of variance that can bias statistical inference. Put another way, conclusions about whether there are statistically significant improvements in health before and after treatment, or between providers, could be affected by the choice of the value set used to summarise patients' data. This is a potentially important issue for routine use of these sorts of data in PROs programmes.

Regardless of which approach is taken to summarising the data, it is important to recognise that patients' responses to *individual question items* are themselves worth scrutinising. The patients' responses to each question can tell us some quite important things about their experience of health problems that can be missed by focusing just on the overall summary scores or values. For example, Gutacker *et al.* (2013b) show that hospitals' performance in improving patient health differed by EQ-5D dimension (this study is described in more detail in Chapter 5). Devlin *et al.* (2010) show some simple ways that EQ-5D profile data can be used to explore changes in patient health, without having to introduce either summary scores or values.

Condition-specific and generic PROs

Given that the condition-specific and generic PROs instruments are clearly very different, is one type better than the other? More generally, on what basis might any given PROs instrument be judged superior to any other?

There is a considerable volume of health services, psychometric, clinical and economics research literature on these issues, but, in brief, generic instruments such as the EQ-5D and SF-36 have been shown to work well in a wide range of health problems. They measure health in ways that:

- are broadly consistent with other, different, ways of measuring health (validity)
- mean individual health experiences tend to be reported in the same way (reliability)
- capture salient changes to health (sensitivity).

However, for some patient groups, and some sorts of health problems, generic instruments do not perform well on these criteria, and seem to miss important aspects of health status and changes in health.

The condition-specific instruments in common use generally do tend to be valid, reliable and sensitive. Usually (although not always) they outperform the generic instruments in capturing the detail of specific conditions. They are more focused on a tightly defined aspect of health, and tend to be good measures of that. However, the measures of health they produce do not allow comparisons of health across patients with different sorts of conditions. This is a fundamental limitation in many of the applications we will discuss.

For these reasons, the usual recommendation, no matter what the application, is that *both* a condition-specific and a generic PRO measure be used, as is the case in the current collection of PRO data in the English NHS PROMs programme. The condition-specific PRO measure provides a detailed picture of a patient's assessment of his or her own health, and is the kind of PRO most likely to be relevant in clinical practice (see Chapter 4). It also helps to check that the generic measure does not miss anything that is important from the patient's perspective. The generic PRO measure provides the vital common currency that allows for aggregation and comparison across completely different patient groups and health services. It is the generic measures that are most relevant in applications such as assessments of value-for-money (see Chapter 6) and analysis of NHS productivity and performance (see Chapter 7).

Subjective health measures

One concern about the use of PRO information that is occasionally noted is that the data are subjective. That is, they rely on patients' views and feelings, with the implication that these are neither an adequate nor appropriate basis for making important decisions.

PRO data *are* subjective – but purposefully so! Their intention is to capture patients' views about their own health on the grounds that making patients feel better and making them better able to do what they want to do – everyday functions – is the goal of most health services, and that patients are usually likely to be the best judge of how they feel.

However, PROs complement rather than replace clinical assessments as information that aids decision-making. For example, raised blood pressure and high cholesterol are extremely important indicators of serious health problems, but because these will not be felt by patients, their presence or alleviation will not be detected by PROs. Occasionally, PROs may pose considerable challenges – relying on patients to self-report their health is difficult with patients suffering from severe cognitive deficits, paralysis or dementia, or those who are unconscious or not literate. There are also clearly problems where an intervention pre-empts the emergence of a condition that would harm a patient's health. While proxy versions of PROs that can be completed by, for example, caregivers and PROs designed for completion by specific groups such as children are available, the reliance on self-reporting health presents an issue for the use of PROs in some contexts.

Measuring changes in health

So far, PROs have been described as measuring patient-reported health at a point in time. But most of the uses of PRO data we will consider involve, in one way or another, measuring and comparing *changes* in health. If the purpose of health care is to improve how patients feel, or to prevent them from feeling worse, then PROs must be used across time, such as before and after treatment, so that it is possible to gauge what improvement or other change has occurred that might be attributable to treatment.

In the current PROMs programme in the English NHS, data are collected before and after each of four elective surgical procedures. In each case, the health care intervention - surgery – is a one-off, well-defined procedure. A simple before-and-after measurement of PROs is most likely to yield helpful information in this situation. Yet even then, what would have happened in the absence of surgery – the counterfactual – remains unknown (for a detailed discussion of this issue, see Chapter 7). Other schemes collect follow-up data for longer periods, for example the UK National Joint Register collects PROs from hip and knee replacement patients at baseline (pre-surgery) and at 6 months, 1 year and 3 years after surgery.

In other situations, the treatment or intervention might be less well defined or more prolonged, and therefore more variable in the quantity and quality of delivery, for example support services, home-help and counselling. The condition might be chronic and the treatment an ongoing process rather than a point-in-time intervention, for example asthma, chronic obstructive pulmonary disease, care and support services for schizophrenia. Also, treatment might be more likely to comprise a complex package of health and social care rather than a single intervention.

These characteristics pose substantial, although not insurmountable, challenges for data collection and analysis, which we address in later chapters.

Ways of summarising and presenting PROs

Presenting PRO data to the public and patients in an unambiguous and comprehensible manner presents a real challenge. However, a prior issue is *what* data or measures to present. For all the PROs in routine use in the NHS, there are many different ways of presenting and summarising the data each measure captures.

For example, patients' EQ-5D profile (their answers to the five sets of questions) can be assigned a social value to produce a single index number scaled between 0 and 1 and then further adjusted to account for case-mix differences. Alternatively, patients' own overall assessment of their health on the 0–100 visual analogue scale (EQ-VAS) can be used. And further, the disease-specific measures such as the Oxford hip and knee score or the Aberdeen Varicose Vein score convey additional information about patients' reported outcomes. But which approach best conveys what patients want to know when it comes to decisions about their treatment or hospital?

Below, we describe some of the ways PRO data can be analysed and presented, drawing on recent research and current recommendations.

Summarising PROs data

The recommendation from the PROMs pilot study commissioned by the Department of Health was that both the generic measure of health – the EQ-5D – and the disease-specific measures should be made available, at the level of hospitals. For the EQ-5D, the recommendation from the pilot PROMs research was that the 'mean post-operative [PROMs] scores adjusted for the value attached to different EQ-5D health states and then further adjusted for patients' pre-operative characteristics' (Browne *et al.* 2007) is the preferred measure of health gain. How the scores are calculated was described earlier.

The use of these values is common practice in economic evaluations, where they are applied to EQ-5D data and used as a means of estimating the 'Q' in QALYs. But is the use of these values appropriate for PROs?

First, these social values come from having asked members of the general public their opinions about EQ-5D states that they may or may not have experienced. The values do not come from patients completing the PROs instruments. This means that the data can no longer be regarded as being purely *patient-reported*, since each patient's score incorporates values that reflect the preferences of the general public about the patient's health state. This can bias conclusions about whether a given change in health is statistically significant (Parkin *et al.* 2010).

Secondly, collapsing the EQ-5D profile data into one score, while potentially useful in many respects, also means losing information about where differences in health are to be found; that is, in which dimensions of health-related quality of life. For example, differences may be due to changes in one particular dimension, which may be worth knowing about.

Thirdly, the recommendation to focus on post-operative EQ-5D data as the measure of interest appears to miss the opportunity to compare the before and after EQ-5D data. In other words, there is no comparison of the *change* in EQ-5D measure. The adjusted health gain measure for each hospital recommended by Browne *et al.* essentially reports the difference between a *predicted* average post-operation EQ-5D score for each hospital (built up from individual patient scores) and the national average pre-operative score. The predicted score takes account of every patients' *pre-operative* score plus a range of patient characteristics used to account for differences in case-mix between hospitals.

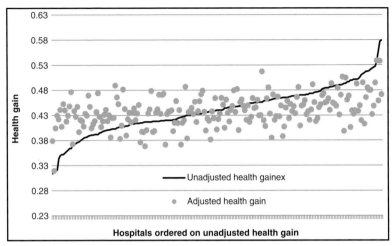

Figure 2.1 Adjusted and unadjusted EQ-5D index scores for primary hip replacement: English hospitals, 2012–2013: ordered on both adjusted and unadjusted results. Source: Data: HSCIC (2014)

While the adjusted health gain score is a valid way of reporting health gain, it is not the same as a straight difference between each hospital's pre and post-operative scores. As Figure 2.1 shows, the impact of the particular case-mix adjustment method produces a range and pattern of health gain across hospitals which seems not too dissimilar to a ranking of unadjusted gains. However, as Figure 2.2 shows, these orderings hide the fact that the adjustment produces a very different ordering of health gain for hospitals as individual hospital's adjusted gains are in many cases considerably different from their unadjusted results.

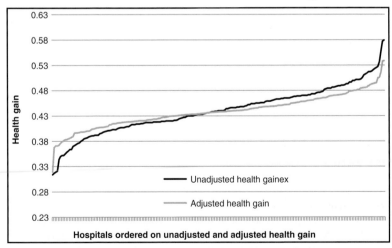

Figure 2.2 Adjusted and unadjusted EQ-5D index scores for primary hip replacement: English hospitals, 2012–2013: ordered on unadjusted results only. Source: Data: HSCIC (2014)

Given these problems, an alternative approach would be to measure in health terms the value added by treatment, that is, to use patients' before and after EQ-5D data to see what difference the provider/treatment made to patient health. However, there is then a question of what constitutes a significant or minimally important difference (MID) in scores.

As Figure 2.1 shows, there is a statistical answer to the meaningful change problem and this is to calculate confidence intervals around the average score to indicate the probability of the score being different simply due to random variations in the data. The average difference between before and after scores for a procedure in one hospital compared with another, for example, would be interpreted as being statistically different if the confidence intervals did not overlap. However, while scores may differ significantly in a statistical sense, such differences may not necessarily be clinically important in the sense that they mean much to patients.

Although there are other ways to identify MIDs, the PROs evaluation carried out for the Department of Health found that across all the PROs measures tested, including the generic and disease-specific measures, it was difficult to pinpoint what might constitute an MID (Browne *et al.*, 2007). While the current recommendation is to use statistical significance testing as a guide to important or meaningful differences there is clearly a need to explore further what changes are important and meaningful to patients.

Categorising changes in the EQ-5D profile

Rather than summarising EQ-5D profiles by their social values an alternative approach is to examine the health profile data itself. One way of doing this is to use an approach developed by Devlin *et al.* (2010): the Paretian Classification of Health Change (PCHC). (Paretian principles are central to welfare economics; they concern the way individual preferences, expressed in ordinal terms, can be aggregated to make social judgements about whether welfare has improved.) This approach is based on the idea of identifying unambiguous improvements or deteriorations, and, specifically, where:

- an improvement means improvement in problems on at least one dimension and no worsening on any other
- a worsening means worsening in the level of problems on at least one dimension and no improvement on any other
- a mixed result means improvement (or worsening) in the level of problems on one or more dimensions and worsening (or improvement) on one or more others.

This has the advantage of revealing a bit more information from the raw EQ-5D profile data, information that can be lost when summarised into a single number. Figure 2.3 gives an example of how such information can be presented, using anonymous patient-level data from the English PROMs programme for 2010–2011.

Disease specific outcome measures

While the EQ-5D represents a useful generic measure of health-related quality of life, and allows comparison, for example, between different types of treatment, disease or procedure-specific measures provide another take on patients' reported outcomes. These have the potential to focus on specific dimensions of outcome – such as pain or mobility – likely to be of particular concern to patients undergoing particular procedures - such as hip replacement.

A question that arises from the bar chart in Figure 2.3 is how and why the disease specific results differ from the generic EQ-5D measure. There is a fairly high degree of concordance for hip and knee replacement disease specific and generic outcome results, but a big difference

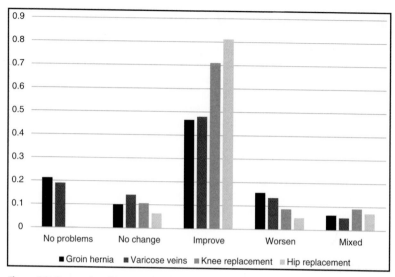

Figure 2.3 Presentation of Paretian Classification of Health Change using EQ-5D profile data before and after four elective procedures. Source: Data: HSCIC (2012)

for varicose veins, with the specific measure reporting a higher level of improvement (84.1%) than the generic measure (39.6%). However, while researchers have shown that while there is good agreement between disease-specific and generic results for major surgery such as hip and knee replacement, the ratings of around 30% of hospitals in the case of hip replacements and 16% in the case of knee replacements varied depending on the choice of outcome measure (Neuberger *et al.*, 2013). One conclusion from this research in terms of which measure to use was whether '...the priority is to avoid missing "poor" providers or avoid mislabelling average providers as "poor"'.

Although the most significant disagreement occurs with two out of four of the procedures examined, it does illustrate the potential confusion for patients in understanding which measure best reflects the truth of patients' subjective assessments.

The question of how the results on disease specific (and generic outcome measures) correlate with other outcomes, such as complications and patient satisfaction, have been explored by researchers. For example, Grosse *et al.* (2012a) found that amongst patients reporting a complication following surgery for hip and knee replacement, hernias and varicose veins, both the disease specific and generic health gain scores were lower than those without complications The same researchers also found that significant improvements in patient satisfaction with surgery correlated well with improvements reported on disease-specific measures, though somewhat less well with generic measures of outcome (Grosse *et al.*, 2012b). As they conclude, including a single question on patient satisfaction can add '...additional insight into the impact of surgery'.

While there is some comfort in the fact that there is some agreement between patient reported and clinical measures of outcome following surgery, it remains too that there are differences. Although this may appear confusing to patients, we should perhaps not expect complete agreement given the different aspects/types of outcome different measures investigate.

Measurement of *overall* health

As part of its generic health measure, the English NHS PROMs initiative collects information on patients' overall health, using a visual analogue scale, the EQ-VAS, where the lower bound, labelled zero is 'worst imaginable health' and 100 is 'best imaginable health'. Comparison of the before and after values on this broad measure provide an alternative indicator of value-added health-related quality of life. An example, for the EQ-VAS reported by patients before and after varicose vein surgery, is shown in Figure 2.4. This shows the percentage of patients for each hospital reporting an improvement or no change or a worsening on the visual analogue scale. Net changes (improvement minus unchanged/worsened – the lighter shades) reveal just five hospitals (out of 53) with an average improvement for their hernia patients as a whole.

Again, however, there remains the problem of what might justifiably constitute an MID on this measure. Furthermore, the PROMs pilot study reported that patients were not particularly enthusiastic about this measure. Presentation of this sort of data could be similar to that for the EQ-5D overall score, using vertical histograms together with confidence intervals.

Funnel plots

The evaluative research for the Department of Health suggested that the mean post-operative EQ-5D score, both unadjusted and adjusted for pre-operative patient characteristics recommended to the Department should be illustrated in the form of funnel plots (see Box 2.4). These can show the summary scores for each hospital plotted against the volume of work carried out in each hospital. However, focus group work with managers, clinicians and patients indicated that 'patients were less enamoured' than commissioners and managers with the use of funnel plots as a way of communicating a PRO summary indicator (Browne *et al.*, 2007).

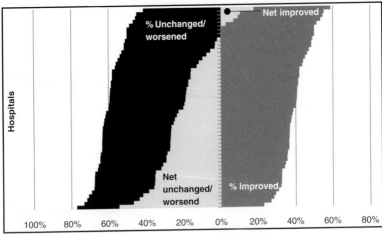

Figure 2.4 EQ-VAS change before and after varicose vein surgery: percentage reporting improvement or unchanged/worsened. English hospitals: April 2012–March 2013. Source: Data: HSCIC (2014)

Box 2.4 What is a funnel plot?

In the context of the reporting of PROMs, a funnel plot is a scatter diagram of the PROMs summary outcome measure for each hospital, plotted against the total number of operations each hospital performed. The tendency is for average PROMs values to vary more widely for those hospitals undertaking fewer operations than those carrying out more. The resulting plots funnel down from left to right.

The funnel plot shows the performance of hospitals measured in terms of the adjusted health gain across all patients undergoing – in this case – a knee replacement between April 2012 and March 2013. Changes in the health measure (the EQ-5D index) are adjusted for various patient factors which vary between hospitals and which may affect the gains in health. This case-mix adjustment allows a better comparison between hospitals.

The horizontal line shows the average health gain for England as a whole (in this case equal to 0.3182). Given random variation in the data, the fact that a hospital's average health gain score falls below this average is not necessarily conclusive proof that the hospital is doing worse than average.

However, if a hospital falls below the lower control limits or above the upper limits then this is a much stronger indication of poor or good performance. Control limits (the dotted lines in the figure) are set at 95 and 98.9%. A hospital at the former limit means that there is a 1 in 20 chance of this simply being a random event; the latter, much tighter control, implies a 1 in 500 chance of the result simply being the outcome of random variation.

It is important to note that while control limits are calculated statistically and become tighter around the average as the number of operations increases, they are essentially based on a judgement about what should and should not be considered acceptable variation in performance.

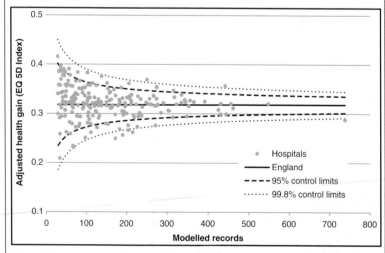

Figure 2.5 Case-mix adjusted average health gain: Primary knee replacement, English hospitals, April 2012–March 2013. Source: Data: HSCIC (2014)

Conclusions

From this primer on PROs it is hopefully clear that there is tremendous scope and potential power in formalising perhaps the most common opening question from a doctor to their patient: 'How are you feeling today?' The questionnaires that have been developed to capture the essence – but also the complexities – of the patient's response to the doctor's inquiry do not of course aim to replace the question. But they do offer a way to quantify and compare patients' answers to this most basic of questions. We go on to look at how patients may (and do) use PROs information next.

There is a large and growing body of evidence and information on patient reported outcomes. Some selected resources are shown in Box 2.5.

Box 2.5 Further resources about patient reported outcome measures

The following web sites provide a handy source of free information, including references to key publications reporting on patient reported outcomes.

The Health and Social Care Information Centre (HSCIC) collates and publishes data from the English NHS PROMs initiative. Information and data can be found here: www.hscic.gov.uk/proms.

Oxford University provide an extensive, searchable database of PRO instruments: www.phi.uhce.ox.ac.uk/.

The EuroQol Group website (www.euroqol.org) provides information on the EQ5D instruments and a searchable reference list. Users of the EQ-5D must register their studies with the EuroQol Group and respect the copyright on the instrument. However, the EQ-5D is generally free-of-charge for academic research use, and NHS users can now also use the EQ-5D under an arrangement with the Department of Health.

Information on the US-based initiative on PROs – 'PROMIS' – is available on this site, www.nihpromis.org/about/abouthome.

The International Society for Pharmacoeconomics and Outcomes Research (ISPOR) provides useful material on patient-reported outcome methods, concepts and studies on its website: www.ispor.org/.

ProQolid (www.proqolid.org/) is the France-based MAPI Institute's database of instruments. This is publicly accessible, with payment options for additional access.

The London School of Hygiene and Tropical Medicine established and maintain a bibliographic database of published and grey literature on research using patient reported outcome measures: http://proms.lshtm.ac.uk/.

References

Alberta Health (2013) *Health System Outcomes and Measurement Framework* [Internet]. Government of Alberta. 2013 [cited 2014 Dec 29]. Available from: www.health.alberta.ca/documents/PMIS-Outcomes-Measurement-Framework-2014.pdf (accessed 15 June, 2015).

Barker K (2014) A new settlement for health and social care: Final Report (The Barker Commission). The King's Fund, London. Available at: www.kingsfund.org.uk/sites/files/kf/field/field_publication_file/Commission%20Final%20interactive.pdf (accessed 15 June, 2015).

Barry MJ, Fowler FJ Jr, O'Leary MP, Bruskewitz RC, Holtgrewe HL, Mebust WK, Cockett AT (1992) The American Urological Association symptom index for benign prostatic hyperplasia. The Measurement Committee of the American Urological Association. *Journal of Urology*, vol 148, no 5, pp 1549–1557; discussion 1564.

Bowling A. (2004) *Measuring Health: A Review of Quality of Life Measurement Scales*, 3rd edition, Maidenhead, UK: Open University Press.

Bowling A. (2001) *Measuring Disease*, 2nd edition, Maidenhead, UK: Open University Press.

Brooks R (1996) EuroQol: the current state of play. *Health Policy*, vol 37, no 1, pp 53–72.

Browne J, Jamieson L, Lewsey J, van der Meulen J, Black N, Cairns J, Lamping D, Smith S, Copley L, Horrocks, J (2007) Patient Reported Outcome Measures (PROMs) in Elective Surgery. *Report to the Department of Health*. London: Health Services Research Unit, London School of Hygiene & Tropical Medicine and Clinical Effectiveness Unit, Royal College of Surgeons of England. Available at: www.lshtm.ac.uk/hsru/research/PROMs-Report-12-Dec-07.pdf (accessed 15 June, 2015).

Cleary PD, Crofton C, Hays RD, Horner R. (2012) Advances from the Consumer Assessment of Healthcare Providers and Systems (CAHPS®) Project. Introduction. *Medical Care*, 2012 Nov, vol 50, Suppl S1. doi: 10.1097/MLR.0b013e31826ec0cb.

Coast J, Flynn N, Natarajan L, Sproston, K, Lewis J, Louviere J, Peters T (2008) Valuing the ICECAP capability index for older people. *Social Science & Medicine*, vol 67, no 5. doi: 10.1016/j.socscimed.2008.05.015.

Dawson J, Fitzpatrick R, Carr A, Murray D. (1996) Questionnaire on the perceptions of patients about total hip replacement. *J Bone Joint Surg Br*, vol 78, no 2, pp 185–190.

Dawson J, Fitzpatrick R, Murray D, Carr A (1998) Questionnaire on the perceptions of patients about total knee replacement. *The Journal of Bone and Joint Surgery, British Volume*, vol 80, no 1, pp 63–69.

Devlin N, Parkin D, Browne J (2010) Patient Reported Outcome Measures in the NHS: new methods for analysing and reporting EQ-5D data. *Health Economics*, vol 19, pp 886–905.

Feng Y, Parkin D, Devlin NJ (2014) Assessing the performance of the EQ-VAS in the NHS PROMs programme. *Quality of Life Research*, vol 23, no 3, pp 977–989. doi: 10.1007/s11136–013–0537-z.

Garratt A, Macdonald L, Ruta D, Russell I, Buckingham JK, Krukowski Z. (1993) Towards measurement of outcome for patients with varicose veins. *Quality in Health Care*, vol 2, pp 5–1.

Grosse Frie K, van der Meulen J, Black N. (2012a) Relationship between patients' reports of complications and symptoms, disability and quality of life after surgery. *Brit J Surg*, 99, 1156–1163.

Grosse Frie K, van der Meulen J, Black N. (2012b) Single item on satisfaction with condition provided additional insight into impact of surgery. *J Clin Epidemiol* 65, pp 619–626.

Gutacker N, Bojke C, Daidone S, Devlin N, Street A. (2013b) Hospital variation in patient reported outcomes at the level of EQ-5D dimensions: evidence from England. *Med Decis Making*, vol 33, no 6, pp 804–818. doi: 10.1177/0272989×13482523.

Hawthorne G, Richardson J, Osborn R (1999) The Assessment of Quality of Life (AQoL) instrument: a psychometric measure of health-related quality of life. *Quality of Life Research*, 8, 209–224.

Health and Social Care Information Centre (2014) *Provisional Monthly Patient Reported Outcome Measures (PROMs) in England – April to March 2013, May 2014 release*. Leeds: HSCIC.

Health and Social Care Information Centre (2012) *PROMs Special Topic, Patient-level Data - 2009–2012*. Available at www.hscic.gov.uk/catalogue/PUB08222 (accessed 15 June, 2015).

Herdman M, Sanz L, Lloyd A, Badia X, Gudex C (2008) Qualitative testing of two new 5-level versions of the EQ-5D in Spain: preliminary study results. Paper presented at the *EuroQol Group Scientific Plenary, Lake Maggiore, Italy*.

Horsman, J., Furlong, W., Feeny, D. and Torrance, G. (2003) The Health Utilities Index (HUI®): concepts, measurement properties and applications. *Health and Quality of Life Outcomes*, 1, 54.

Kharroubi SA, Brazier JE, Roberts J, O'Hagan A. (2007) Modelling SF-6D health state preference data using a nonparametric Bayesian method. *Journal of Health Economics*, vol 26, pp 597–612.

Morris S, Devlin N, Parkin D, Spencer A (2012) *Economic Analysis in Health Care*, 2nd Edition. Chichester: John Wiley & Sons, Ltd.

National Institute for Health and Care Excellence (2013) *Guide to the Methods of Technology Appraisal 2013*. Available at: http://publications.nice.org.uk/pmg9 (accessed 15 June, 2015).

Netten A, Burge P, Malley J, Potoglou D, Towers A, Brazier J, Flynn T, Forder J, Wall B (2012) Outcomes of Social Care for Adults: Developing a Preference-Weighted Measure, *Health Technology Assessment*, vol 16, no 16, pp 1–165. http://dx.doi.org/10.3310/hta16160.

Neuburger J, Hutchings A, van der Meulen J, Black N (2013) Using patient reported outcomes (PROs) to compare the performance of providers: does the choice of measure matter? *Medical Care*, vol 51, pp 517–523.

O'Boyle C (1994) Schedule for the Evaluation of Individual Quality of Life (SEIQOL) *Int. J. Ment. Health*, vol 23, no 3, pp 3–23.

Parkin D, Rice N, Devlin N. (2010) Statistical analysis of EQ-5D profiles: does the use of value sets bias inference? *Medical Decision Making*, Vol. 30, no. 5, pp 556–565.

Steinberg EP, Tielsch JM, Schein OD, Javitt JC, Sharkey P, Cassard SD, Legro MW, Diener-West M, Bass EB, Damiano AM, et al. (1994) The VF-14. An index of functional impairment in patients with cataract. *Archives of Ophthalmology*, vol 112, no 5, pp 630–638.

Szende A, Janssen, B, Cabases, J (eds) (2014) *Measuring self-reported population health: Self-Reported Population Health: An International Perspective based on EQ-5D*. Dordrecht, The Netherlands: Springer.

Szende A, Oppe M, Devlin N (eds) (2007) *EQ-5D Value Sets: Inventory, Comparative Review and User Guide*. EuroQol Group monographs volume 2. Dordrecht, The Netherlands: Springer.

Walters AS, LeBrocq C, Dhar A, Hening W, Rosen R, Allen RP, Trenkwalder C; International Restless Legs Syndrome Study Group (2003) Validation of the International Restless Legs Syndrome Study Group rating scale for restless legs syndrome. *Sleep Medicine*, vol 4, no 2, pp 121–132.

Ware JE Jr, Sherbourne CD (1992) The MOS 36-item short-form health survey (SF-36). I. Conceptual framework and item selection. *Medical Care*, vol 30, no 6, pp 473–483.

WHOQOL Group. (1998) The World Health Organization quality of life assessment (WHOQOL): Development and general psychometric properties. *Social Science and Medicine*, vol 46, no 12, pp 1569–1585.

CHAPTER 3

Patients: information and choice

Patients are not only the source of PRO data, but also a key potential user of the information they generate. Patients suffering from health problems and being considered for treatment will be able to refer to the PRO data provided by similar sorts of patients to help them:

- judge the likely benefits of treatment in their own case.
- decide where and from whom to receive treatment.

Here we consider the various ways in which PRO data could be – and is – used by patients.

Patient choice

Enhancing patient choice has been a key theme in English health policy reform and is part of a wider goal of increasing the responsiveness of the NHS to patients' preferences. This has been particularly reflected in a shift towards offering patients who need a hospital referral a choice about which hospital they attend.

Specific NHS patient choice initiatives in England started with the London Patient Choice Project in 2002, which was followed by the national choice initiatives for coronary heart disease. In 2005 patient choice was extended to all NHS patients in England who were being referred to hospital, giving them a choice of five providers. Since 2008, NHS patients in England have been offered an open choice of any NHS, and some independent sector, providers in England.

As patient choice of provider has been rolled out across the NHS, a growing body of research and experience has accumulated about how patients make choices about their hospital, and the sort of information patients say is important to them in making those choices.

To date, information for patients on hospital performance has generally been limited to indicators of negative outcomes, such as rates of post-operative mortality, readmission and methicillin-resistant *Staphylococcus aureus* (MRSA) infection, which are relevant in only a minority of cases. The introduction of PROs is, in part, a response to the need to provide better information to patients about provider performance in improving health. But how will patients use this information? How is it most effectively presented to patients? Will the availability of PRO data change their choices? And how will providers respond? In particular, given the variety of PRO data – the EQ-5D index, the visual analogue score, the disease-specific measures as well as the often complex ways these can be presented – which will patients find potentially useful information, and which too confusing to use?

Using Patient Reported Outcomes to Improve Health Care,
First Edition. John Appleby, Nancy Devlin and David Parkin.
© 2016 John Wiley & Sons, Ltd. Published 2016 by John Wiley & Sons, Ltd.

Which treatment?

Although the main focus of national policy on patient choice in the English NHS has been on choice of hospital, there are, of course, more fundamental choices that patients have to confront, not the least of which is choosing whether to have any medical treatment at all, and if so, which of various treatment options that might be available.

The guidelines on informed consent issued by the General Medical Council (GMC; *see* Box 3.1) make it clear that doctors are required to provide a range of information about treatment options for patients including: 'The potential benefits, risks and burdens, and the likelihood of success, for each option; *this should include information, if available, about whether the benefits or risks are affected by which organisation or doctor is chosen to provide care*' (our emphasis) (General Medical Council, 2008, paragraph 9, sub-section (e), p. 10).

Box 3.1 GMC guidelines on informed consent

9. [Doctors] must give patients the information they want or need about:
   a. the diagnosis and prognosis
   b. any uncertainties about the diagnosis or prognosis, including options for further investigations
   c. options for treating or managing the condition, including the option not to treat
   d. the purpose of any proposed investigation or treatment and what it will involve
   e. the potential benefits, risks and burdens, and the likelihood of success, for each option; this should include information, if available, about whether the benefits or risks are affected by which organisation or doctor is chosen to provide care
   f. whether a proposed investigation or treatment is part of a research programme or is an innovative treatment designed specifically for their benefit
   g. the people who will be mainly responsible for and involved in their care, what their roles are, and to what extent students may be involved
   h. their right to refuse to take part in teaching or research
   i. their right to seek a second opinion
   j. any bills they will have to pay
   k. any conflicts of interest that you, or your organisation, may have
   l. any treatments that you believe have greater potential benefit for the patient than those you or your organisation can offer.

Source: General Medical Council (2008, p 10).

There are two important issues regarding this aspect of the GMC guidance. First, it notes that patients should be given information about the benefits and risks of any treatment option. Second, it also instructs doctors to tell patients if such benefits/risks vary by hospital or clinician.

PROs information can play a supporting role in helping doctors and patients with making informed treatment choices. At present, on their own, PRO data do not have the power to predict the benefits (or lack of them) of a particular treatment option for a particular patient. However, as the NHS in England accumulates data on PROs, there is the potential to establish, via risk adjustment, the extent to which certain patient characteristics – such as age, sex, pre-existing conditions, severity of condition and so on – are associated with changes in PROs (see Box 3.2).

Box 3.2 Initial investigation of data collected by the NHS as part of the PROMS pilot study

A study of 410 patients who underwent a hip replacement operation examined whether a range of factors relating to patient and clinical characteristics were associated with the outcomes of surgery (Devlin et al., 2010). The factors examined included the pre-operative disease-specific health measure (the Oxford Hip and Knee Score), sex, symptom duration, co-morbidities, a composite score of socioeconomic deprivation, and a general measure of health and hospital.

The study examined whether these factors could be used to predict the probability of patients showing, following surgery, as measured by the EQ-5D:

- improvement (on at least one dimension, with no worsening on any other)
- worsening (on at least one dimension, with no improvement on any other)
- mixed change (improvement on one or more dimensions, worsening on one or more dimensions).

Overall, the patient's pre-operative health and other factors were poor at explaining changes in the EQ-5D, due in part to the small numbers involved. However, the pre-operative measure was significant and suggested that patients with a worse score on this measure had a higher probability of improvement post-operatively as measured by the PROM EQ-5D. Age and sex, on the other hand, appeared to be unrelated to the change in the EQ-5D measure.

This study was small-scale and no robust conclusions can be drawn. However, it shows how, as more PROMs data are collected, the relationships between PROMs information and other factors can be investigated.

Similarly, comparative PRO data at hospital (and clinician) level can provide patients with an insight into any outcome variations that might exist.

An example of the active use of PRO data to help patients in their choices is the use of outcome data in general practice as part of initial consultations between patients and their GPs. Box 3.3 details the experience of one English GPs' use of PRO data in consultations with his patients. The impact on his patients' decisions about whether to undergo surgery for their hernias is perhaps surprising. We look at some the issues raised here from the point of view of the clinician in the next chapter.

Box 3.3 The use of PROMs data in general practice consultations

Dr Tim Hughes is a GP practising in Kirkbymoorside on the southern edge of the North York Moors. Since the summer of 2013 Dr Hughes has been using data on patient reported outcomes of groin hernia and other interventions in his consultations with patients.

How did you know about PROMs?

Professor Alan Maynard is chairman of my local Clinical Commissioning Group and he introduced me to the PROMs data that was being collected in English hospitals since 2009. I thought this is a goldmine on information! Now my partners and registrars are starting to use the PROMs data as part of the process of shared decision making.

What PROM data do you show patients?

We use the information available on the NHS Choices website; there is a link to the main PROMs data site where there is a summary graph of the four procedures currently covered by PROMs. I've printed the graph off, laminated it and have it in the consulting room! (See Figure 3.1 and Appendix 3.) I explain the terminology to patients – the Oxford Hip Score, the EQ-5D Index and so on – and people very quickly look at the figures and see that, especially in the case of hernias and varicose veins, a lot of people felt worse after their operation. My patients are surprised by that.

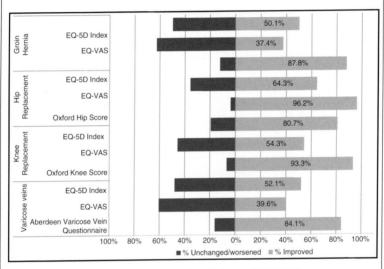

Figure 3.1 PROMs outcomes: April 2012–March 2013. Source: HSCIC (2014)

Are hospital specialists using PROMs data?

There is one surgeon in my area who has started using PROMs data in his outpatient clinics. He has told me that he had seen a patient referred from another practice and shown them some of the PROMs data on hernias. Partly on the basis of the patient reported outcomes the patient decided not to have an operation but to wait and monitor how they felt, how much pain they were in and so on. I thought this is great, a surgeon using the PROMs data with a patient and not operating! Unfortunately, I think most surgeons won't do that; they just want to operate.

How do patients react when they see the data?

When I show people the PROMS data, they tend to weigh up how they currently feel (in terms of pain and the things they can and cannot do) against the possible costs of the operation leaving them worse off.

The PROMs data changes patients' perceptions. People look at the data and they're surprised by the hernia feedback because they think that an operation should make you better. I have to say that it was a real surprise to me too about how many people felt worse after their hernia operations. It was a shock actually, because patients are very grateful for what they get and they don't tell you when things aren't so good – they just put up with it. They may feel that it's a bit painful now, but perhaps expect that it will get better. And of course it often doesn't.

It's useful to have the different procedures together for comparison too, with the hips and knees and varicose veins results all together. People look at that these as well and note how good a hip operation seems to be. Seeing the results for the other conditions gives them confidence in the hernia information.

They also, of course, know their own experience. People really value the experience of others. They ask other people how they felt about their operations. They might say, 'My mate didn't really think it helped him very much' – but then think that was only one person's view about their own experience. But when they see thousands of people saying the same thing, then they think again.

What has been the impact of PROMs data on patients' decisions about treatment?
I think there has been a general perception that, even if there was a low risk of obstruction with a hernia it was worth referring a patient for an operation. Also, there has been a general opinion that it would be better to have an operation at younger ages. So, I think there has been a tendency to refer patients to specialists and to let the consultant decide what to do. But surgeons want to operate – so everyone gets operated on! But the PROMs results now emerging are changing that.

When I started using the PROMs data as part of informed decision making with patients, of the seven people in six months who had inguinal hernias, none were referred to specialists at the initial consultation. One patient was referred later because he was in pain all the time so thought he would go ahead with the operation – even if there was a risk of a poor outcome.

So, instead of the decision to operate being made in the hospital with a surgeon (who will have a natural bias towards operating rather than not operating) the decision is being made at the consultation with the GP. The information the patient wanted to help them make a decision – will this help me? Will the operation make me better? – is now available from the GP. The PROMs data is very powerful – it changes the consultation because we're both looking at it together and chatting about it.

What effect has the PROMs data had patients with varicose veins?
My CCG inherited a policy view that varicose vein surgery was a procedure of limited clinical value, and hence discouraged referrals. So the discussion I have with patients with varicose veins is different as the choice for them is private treatment. This time, when they see the rather poor PROMs data on varicose veins the decision for them is sharpened somewhat by the fact that it is their own money at stake. They tend to think that they're not likely to get much bang for their buck and I think that the PROMs data has put people off seeing a surgeon privately.

What new developments would you like to see for PROMs?

At the moment we only have PROMs data routinely collected for four procedures. We need this extended to other common interventions too - cataract surgery and the peripheral vascular type of procedures where there is research evidence that such work is perhaps not that effective. But I think we really need PROMs for cardiology procedures as there is a lot of procedures undertaken and I'm not sure we really known the extent to which patients' benefit or not.

PROMs data needs to be much more accessible – physically, and in terms of the clarity of explanations for the measures used. They also need to be much clearer in terms of presentations that patients can understand; the bar graph (see Figure 3.1) is good. But there are other ways of showing this sort of information that we GPs already use – such as the 'hundred smiley faces' (ref www.nntonline.net/) used to convey risk scores to our patients.

It would be very helpful too to have PROMs data easily accessible on our computer systems so we can show it to our patients in a similar way as we currently do with the risks and benefits of, for example, statins. With the statins risks we can quickly show patients how many people out of a hundred may get a heart attack and so on. These are figures and presentations that I find patients really understand. We could do the same with the PROMs data.

Which hospital?

One of the outcomes of Dr Tim Hughes' use of PRO data with his hernia patients was to change their minds about a referral to hospital and the near certainty of an operation; 'watching and waiting' rather than risk a poor surgical outcome seemed preferable. But many people will choose to seek specialist advice and the possibility (or indeed certainty) of further treatment. Such decisions present further choices for patients, such as which hospital to go to.

How patients choose hospitals and the sorts of factors and information they may use to make choices has become increasingly important over the last decade or so as the NHS in England has pursued a more active policy to encourage patient choice. From April 2013 for example, a national roll out of the Friends and Family Test (FFT) started to provide prospective patients with a recommendation metric based on feedback from patients (NHS Choices, 2015a). The FFT results – a score based on the extent to which patients would recommend the hospital they attended to friends and family – are published monthly at the level of wards and hospitals. While fairly straightforward to understand, the FFT approach (akin to the Net Promoter Score used by some private sector businesses as a quick summarised guide to customer satisfaction) has been criticised.

Over the last few years, patients and the public have also been able to 'star rate' NHS hospitals via the NHS Choices website (NHS Choices, 2015b) and leave comments and ratings on individual hospital web sites. This Trip Adviser approach to rating the quality of a hospital has the advantage that it is patient/public-based, but the disadvantage that it also just represents the views of a self-selecting group. Nevertheless, the solicitation and publication of patients' feedback on their experience of NHS services has reflected the widespread use of consumer feedback in many other areas of economic life. But is any of this information useful, or indeed used? And what types of information are most valuable? We have already seen that information reported by patients on changes in their health-related quality of life seems to be important to other patients in consultation with their GP when considering whether or not to have treatment at all, but other factors are likely to be important too when choosing a hospital.

In fact, various surveys and research have confirmed the importance of the quality of a hospital's care in shaping patients' choices. Research carried out in 2005, for example, asked a sample of the public how important factors such as waiting times and hospital facilities were in informing their choice of hospital (Burge *et al.*, 2006). The results, shown in Figure 3.2, suggest, as might be expected, that advice from GPs and waiting times were important to many people in making a choice of hospital. However, the most important factor, with nearly 80% of respondents rating it as very important, was 'the impact on their health as a result of treatment'.

More sophisticated ways of finding out what the public thinks about which aspects of hospitals' services and treatments are important to them have shown that quality of care is paramount. For example, research using a discrete choice experiment (DCE) asked members of the public to choose a hospital for treatment from a list of hospitals with varying performance on, for example waiting times, the impact the hospital would have on their health and other factors such as what their GP advised and travel distances. This work revealed that people weigh up many factors in making a choice: what GPs say about a hospital is influential and waiting times and other factors all play a part in arriving at a decision to go to a particular hospital (Burge *et al.*, 2006).

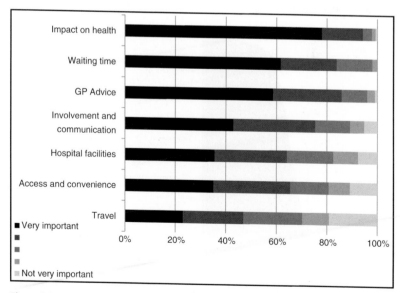

Figure 3.2 Importance of various factors to patients in choosing a hospital for treatment. Source: Burge *et al.* (2006)

The research also showed that trade-offs were made. In an ideal world, patients would want a high-quality hospital on their doorstep with minimal waiting times. However, faced with a less than ideal world, in which waiting times at a local hospital may be longer than those at one that is more distant, for example, people make decisions that reveal the importance of one factor over another. On this basis, 'impact on health' was the most important influence guiding the choices made.

Ironically, at the time the work by Burge *et al.* was carried out the questionnaires designed for the research had to invent a measure for 'impact on health' as no actual measure was in use in the NHS at the time. Since then the English NHS PROMs has provided patient feedback on precisely the information – 'impact on health' – that people said they needed as part of their decision about which hospital to choose.

While Dr Hughes' patients were surprised at the fact that on average around half of those who had an operation for their hernia felt their health related quality of life had either worsened or remained unchanged, they might be even more surprised to learn that the patient reported outcomes from different hospitals varies substantially.

Figure 3.3 for example, ranks 183 English hospitals, both public and private (with patients at the latter paid for by the NHS) between April 2012 and March 2013 according to the proportion of hernia patients reporting an improvement or a worsening/no change in their health. Patients' change in health is based on the difference in pre- and post-operative scores derived from the EQ-5D questionnaire and adjusted to reflect the case-mix of each hospital. Hospitals with fewer than 30 PRO reports are excluded for statistical reasons.

Although the average for all hospitals suggests that around half of those who had an operation reported an improvement in their health, at the extremes this ranged from 28% to 83%. While we cannot be sure whether knowing about this variation would have changed the decisions taken by Dr Hughes' patients, the fact that some hospitals seem to achieve

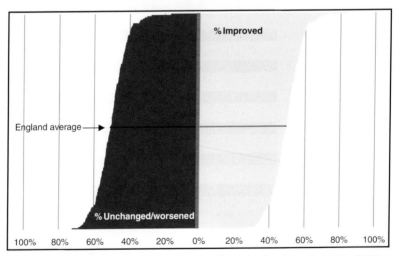

Figure 3.3 Changes in reported health related quality of life for hernia patients: England, April 2012–March 2013 by hospital of treatment. Source: Data: HSCIC (2014). NB: Overall number of patients returning PRO data: 19 372.

substantially better results than others should certainly prompt some further questions for patients. Not least would be the extent to which these outcomes are an accurate prediction for a particular patient. What are the chances that if one of Dr Hughes' patients chose to go to the top performing hospital that they would be one of the 83% reporting an improvement and not one of the 17% who felt worse or had no change in their health? This is a hard question to answer and begs the further question of how the hospital with the best patient reported outcomes achieved such results. Was it, for instance, simply a chance result? Or did the outcomes just reflect a particular group of patients who, because of their particular characteristics (their age, their general levels of health etc.), would have done well no matter which hospital they went to? Or was it to do with other, hospital-related factors such as cleanliness levels, nursing skills and experience? Answering these questions requires further research. However, some of the uncertainty about the results can, to a degree, be addressed.

For example, adjusting each hospital's outcomes to deal with differences in patient characteristics (case-mix adjustment) – as the data in Figure 3.3 have been – helps make the results between hospitals more comparable. Nevertheless, such adjustments cannot rule out completely the chance that the variation between hospital outcomes will to some degree reflect factors related to patients rather than hospitals. Whether the outcomes in Figure 3.3 were simply a matter of chance can also be, again to some degree, addressed statistically. For example, while the outcomes for most of the hospitals in Figure 3.3 were statistically no different from the national average, based on the number of PROs records and the health gain achieved, we can say that the results for the top performing hospital were significantly different from the national average, with less than a 1 in 20 chance of this not being the case.

However, the best performing hospital in the year from April 2012 to March 2013 is one of just 7 (4%) of hospitals that we can say are statistically significantly better than the national average in terms of the average health gain recorded by the EQ-5D PRO measure. And because of the relatively low numbers of reports, we can also say that just 5 (3%) hospitals have results which are significantly worse than the national average. This leaves 172 (93%) which, while their health outcomes vary, *statistically* are likely to be no different from the national average (and hence no different between themselves). The hard statistical conclusion seems to be that even though there are some identifiably good and bad hospitals, most achieve pretty much the same levels of health gain for patients undergoing surgery.

There is a similar level of uncertainty for the EQ-5D results for patients undergoing hip replacements. Figure 3.4 shows that 83% of hospitals are statistically little different from the national average.

The fact that most hospitals appear to achieve similar outcomes is not just a reflection of their actual performance but also simply a technical issue to do with the relatively low number of observations for each hospital. In other words, there may well be real and significant differences in outcomes between hospitals which are being hidden by the data.

One solution to the wide uncertainty caused by relatively low numbers of reports would be to pool data across years, as in Figure 3.5. This is only illustrative and assumes that the health gains and distribution within hospitals of those gains between patients for 2012–2013 were the same for the preceding three years. All that has changed between Figures 3.4 and 3.5 is that the total number of PROs reports (122 740) for the 4 years between 2009 and 2013 have been have been distributed across hospitals in proportion to their 2012–2013 record numbers. Increasing the number of observations shrinks the statistical uncertainty and reveals more hospitals as (statistically) significantly better or worse than the national average.

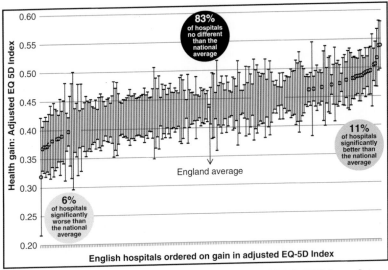

Figure 3.4 Health gain following hip replacement by hospital: England (2012–2013). Source: Data: HSCIC (2014)

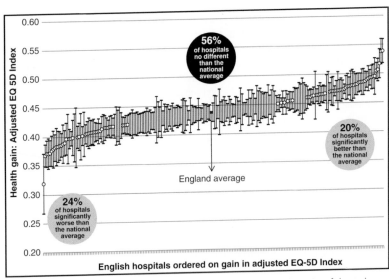

Figure 3.5 Health gain following hip replacement: England, 2012–2013: Illustration of change in confidence intervals with increasing data. Source: Data: HSCIC (2014). NB: The total number of PROs reports (122 740) for the 4 years between 2009 and 2013 have been have been distributed across hospitals in proportion to their 2012–2013 record numbers.

In theory then, pooling the PRO data across years could reveal more statistically valid differences in outcomes between hospitals and hence a better basis to inform patients in their choices about hospitals.

But there's a problem with pooling the data. If hospitals were reasonably consistent performers, generally getting similar outcomes for their patients from year to year, then pooling data across years would be useful and help reveal statistically more meaningful results. Unfortunately, data from England's PROMs programme shows that performance is not necessarily consistent.

Table 3.1 for example, shows hospitals ranked in the top ten each year between 2009 and 2013 in terms of their average adjusted health gain (as measured by the difference between pre and post-operative EQ-5D index scores) for hernia operations. Only three hospitals feature more than once in the top 10 and then in only 2 of the 4 years. Different hospitals fare differently from year to year. Central Manchester – which, out of 157 hospitals had the largest average health gain in 2009–2010, fell to 68th (out of 169) the next year and by 2013–2014 had fallen to 140th (out of 184[2]). The George Eliot hospital has had a more erratic record: second best in 2009–2010 to sixth worst in 2010–2011 and then sixth best in 2011–2012. Pooling PRO data across years may provide a more statistically robust picture of a hospital's performance but at the same time it will hide what patients may feel is important information about trends in performance from year to year.

Table 3.1 Top 10 hospitals by health gain (EQ-5D) for hernia operations: 2009–2010 to 2012–2013

Rank	2009–2010	2010–2011	2011–2012	2012–2013
1	Central Manchester University Hospitals	Claremont Hospital	Homerton University Hospital	BMI : The Foscote Hospital
2	**George Eliot Hospital**	**Nuffield Health: Leicester Hospital**	South Warwickshire	Pinehill Hospital
3	The Midlands NHS Treatment Centre	Dartford and Gravesham	BMI: Goring hill	Nuffield Health: Wolverhampton Hospital
4	Boston NHS Treatment Centre	Great Western Hospitals	Bodmin NHS Treatment centre	Spire: Southampton hospital
5	Royal United Hospital Bath	Northern Lincolnshire and Goole Hospitals	Trafford Health care	BMI: The Chiltern Hospital
6	**Will Adams NHS Treatment Centre**	County Durham and Darlington	**George Eliot Hospital**	Ashford and St Peter's Hospitals
7	Epsom and St Helier University Hospitals	BMI: Bath Clinic	BMI: The Harbour hospital	Wye Valley
8	North Cumbria University Hospitals	BMI: The Beaumont Hospital	Luton and Dunstable university Hospital	Oaks Hospital
9	South London Health care	Dorset County Hospital	**Will Adams NHS Treatment Centre**	SPIRE: Dunedin Hospital
10	Nottingham University Hospitals	Wrightington, Wigan and Leigh	**Nuffield Health: Leicester Hospital**	Nuffield Health: North Staffordshire hospital

Source: Data: HSCIC (2014)

[2] The base number of hospitals varies from year to year depending on – amongst other things – the outcome of the cut off of a minimum of 30 observations per hospital to be included in the outcomes data.

Despite adjustments to the data and the use of statistical tests of significance, it is impossible to eradicate or account for all the uncertainties in the PRO data. Hospital level PRO data can also overturn some patients' certainties – not least that all hospitals are broadly similar in terms the results they achieve. Nevertheless, judgement about the usefulness of PROs should be based not on how far short it falls in providing absolute certainty, but by how much it helps patients make more informed decisions about their care. And it is clear that there is more to understand about the data; the fact that hospital performance varies from year to year is obviously unhelpful for patients and the choices they make. But it should certainly prompt questions for hospitals themselves about the reasons for such inconsistency.

Which clinician?

Of course, patients are not treated by hospitals, and from a patients' point of view knowing the performance of a hospital as a whole is not necessarily as helpful as knowing about individual clinical teams or indeed individual clinicians. And research evidence suggests that patients would overwhelmingly like information on health outcomes not just for hospitals, but at more detailed levels, such as the clinical team that would be involved in their care or individual clinicians (Burge et al., 2006).

While patients in England have had since 2009 a formalised legal right to choose the hospital where they would like to be treated, from April 2012 patients also had a legal right to choose the consultant specialist they would like to see at their first outpatient appointment. As part of an initiative to support patients in their choice of consultant an increasing amount of information is now being made available on key outcomes of treatment by named consultant So far, this data generally includes case-mix adjusted mortality rates and the number of operations for each consultant for ten surgical areas – from cardiac and vascular surgery to urological and colorectal surgery (NHS Choices, 2015c).

Although the publication of mortality data by named surgeon is a significant advance, death within a month (or in some cases 90 days) of an operation is a relatively crude measure of outcome – particularly given its rarity). Death aside, of more relevance to patients would be the impact of an operation by a particular surgeon and their team on their quality of life the sort of information collected by PRO measures such as the EQ-5D and Oxford Hip and Knee Scores can reveal.

As with hospital level reporting of PRO data, there are a number of statistical issues that would need to be dealt with at the individual clinician level too. As with hospital data, there is a need to adjust individual clinician PRO data to standardise as far as possible for variations in patient characteristics. Also, PRO data at the level of a doctor starts to get spread very thinly and, as we have shown for hospital level information, there is a potential problem of lacking enough numbers to make any meaningful comparisons. For example, in the year ending March 2013, there were 30 968 usable PROs records collected across England from patients who had had a hip replacement. While this meant an average of around 150 records per hospital, with approximately 2100 orthopaedic surgeons working in these hospitals the average number of PROs records per surgeon was roughly 15 – a number too small on which to safely basis comparisons. One obvious solution to this low number problem is to boost the numbers by adding years of data together. Over the four years since PROs were collected in England, this would boost the average number of observations per orthopaedic consultant to around 60 and make comparisons between consultants more (statistically) meaningful.

But it is inevitable that, as with pooling data on whole hospitals, pooling consultant level data will obscure trends in the data that might be useful – an erratic performance, or one that has been declining over the years for example.

There is no simple answer to the pooling problem, but as with the recent initiatives to publish surgeon level data on even rarer outcomes – mortality following surgery – there are ways to identify outliers at least by presenting data as funnel plots and choosing agreed limits to identify good, acceptable and poor performance. We discuss this approach and other ways of presenting PRO data next.

Will PROs make a difference to patients' choices?

As noted earlier, surveys show that patients value information on the quality of care impact of treatment on their health to be one of the most important factors when choosing between providers.

Facilitating choice by providing that information was an important reason for the introduction of the PROMs programme in the NHS in England. However, recent research on the impact of patient choice policies on how patients choose, and how providers respond, suggests that in reality patients make limited use of the data already available on hospital characteristics. A survey of nearly 6000 NHS patients in 2009 found:

> Patients drew on various information sources to help them choose, including their own past experience (41 per cent), and advice from their GP (36 per cent) and from friends and family members (18 per cent). Only 4 per cent had looked at the NHS Choices website and 1 per cent consulted other websites.

> Of patients who were offered a choice, 60 per cent were satisfied with the amount of information they were given, 22 per cent did not want any information and 14 per cent would have liked more. (Robertson and Dixon, 2009)

The survey also found that, similar to the studies referred to earlier, cleanliness, quality of care and the standard of facilities were the three most important factors that patients said had influenced their choice of hospital. However, it seems that few patients actively seek and compare the objective information on these factors that is already provided, relying instead on GP recommendations and reputational evidence from friends and family. The relatively poor use by patients of current performance information might, though, reflect their view that this is not the information they really need to make an informed decision.

But it might also reflect the context of the decision facing patients. Dr Tim Hughes' use of PRO data in his consultations with patients was not in the context of choice of hospital but rather more fundamental choice of treatment or no treatment – or rather, treatment or watchful waiting for people with a hernia. What is very interesting about the (albeit small) sample of patients Dr Hughes has involved, is the reaction and eventual decision patients have taken based, in part on the PRO data for hernia outcomes, and in the context of their consultation with their GP. Clearly there is a need to explore in much more detail the use of PRO data as part of shared decision making, but there seems considerable potential in helping to address patients' perennial question – 'What are my chances, Doc?'[3]

[3] In the case of Dr Hughes' hernia patients the answer from the PROMs data seems to be a 50/50 chance of improvement post-surgery – a chance most patients seem to reject as not high enough to warrant the operation.

References

Burge, P, Devlin, N, Appleby J, Gallo F, Nason E, Ling T (2006) *Understanding Patients' Choices at the Point of Referral*. Technical report TR359-DOH. Cambridge: RAND Europe. Available at: www.rand.org/pubs/technical_reports/TR359/ (accessed on 15 June, 2015).

Devlin N, Parkin D, Browne J (2010) Patient Reported Outcome Measures in the NHS: new methods for analysing and reporting EQ-5D data *Health Economics*, vol 19, pp 886–905.

General Medical Council (2008) *Consent: Patients and Doctors Making Decisions Together*. London: General Medical Council. Available at: www.gmc-uk.org/guidance/ethical_guidance/consent_guidance_index.asp (accessed on 1 July 2015).

Health and Social Care Information Centre (2014) *Provisional Monthly Patient Reported Outcome Measures (PROMs) in England – April to March 2013, May 2014 release*. Leeds: HSCIC.

Health and Social Care Information Centre (2012) PROMs Special Topic, Patient-level Data - 2009–2012. Available at www.hscic.gov.uk/catalogue/PUB08222 (accessed 15 June, 2015).

NHS Choices (2015a) The NHS friends and family test. NHS Choices, London. Available at: www.nhs.uk/NHSEngland/AboutNHSservices/Pages/nhs-friends-and-family-test.aspx(accessed 15 June, 2015).

NHS Choices (2015b) NHS Choices: Home page. Available at: www.nhs.uk/Pages/HomePage.aspx (accessed 15 June, 2015).

NHS Choices (2015c) Consultant outcome data. Available at: www.nhs.uk/choiceinthenhs/yourchoices/consultant-choice/pages/consultant-data.aspx.(accessed 15 June, 2015).

Robertson R, Dixon A (2009) *Choice at the Point of Referral: Early results of a patient survey*. Available at: www.kingsfund.org.uk/sites/files/kf/choice-point-of-referral-patient-survey-ruth-robertson-anna-dixon-kings-fund-november-2009.pdf (accessed on 1 July 2015).

CHAPTER 4

Clinicians: clinical decision making

Many clinicians are sceptical about PROs; many others have long been interested in them and some strongly advocate their use in clinical practice. They believe that PROs provide data that make a valuable contribution to their clinical practice and the pursuit of clinical quality.

In 2004, predating the NHS PROMs programme, two of the authors surveyed the Royal Colleges to gauge clinicians' views and practices in this area (Appleby and Devlin, 2004), and were struck by how many examples they found of clinicians collecting and actively using these data to monitor and inform their own clinical practice. These included:

- examining patient PRO data before treatment and using them as a basis for discussing treatment options with patients
- *ad hoc* outcomes-based research on clinical interventions, helping to answer the questions: What works? What does not work?
- obtaining a detailed understanding of how clinical indicators relate to patients' self-reported health.

As reimbursement of providers becomes increasingly linked, either directly through initiatives such as Commissioning for Quality and Innovation (CQUIN; NHS England, 2014) or indirectly via patient choice, to performance on PROs, it is likely that providers will, in turn, wish to use incentives to ensure that the health professionals they employ – who have the most detailed understanding of the factors that lead to improved patient-reported health – are rewarded for good performance. Financial rewards, for example bonuses, may be introduced for exceptional performance or PROs could become part of the evidence used to inform consultants' clinical excellence awards.

Similarly, PROs might be used to identify and address poor performance. Outliers – in terms of lower-than-expected improvements on PROs – could help clinicians to identify poor clinical practices within their own clinical units. PROs could form part of the evidence considered as part of clinicians' annual appraisals and 5-yearly revalidation (Appleby and Devlin, 2004). In extreme cases, PRO data might conceivably be used as part of disciplinary proceedings.

In the NHS PROMs programme, it is possible to link PRO data to individual clinicians through the patient hospital record system (hospital episode statistics – HES). Since late 2012 it is also possible for hospitals to sign up for a service that allows individual clinicians to access individual patient PROMs records for use in their clinical care. Patients are able to grant consent for this sort of use as part of their general consent in completing PROMs questionnaires. But such data will not facilitate the sorts of patient-level uses of PROs that are the focus of this chapter. The use of PROs as a screening tool, a guide to referral, or a means of monitoring and managing patients, will require separate data-collection efforts at the level of the practice itself.

Using Patient Reported Outcomes to Improve Health Care,
First Edition. John Appleby, Nancy Devlin and David Parkin.
© 2016 John Wiley & Sons, Ltd. Published 2016 by John Wiley & Sons, Ltd.

In this chapter, we consider the use of PROs in two aspects of clinical decision making. First, we discuss how condition-specific PROs can be used in clinical practice to benefit patients directly. Second, and rather more controversially, we consider whether there is any place for using PRO data to inform referral practices, for example as part of referral guidelines.

Using PROs in clinical practice

The evidence about the use of PROs in clinical practice is at present still mainly accumulating rather than enabling definitive answers to be given about how, when and where they are most valuable. In a systematic review, Valderas et al. (2008) suggested four potential uses of PROs in daily clinical practice:

- helping to detect health problems that might otherwise be overlooked
- monitoring disease progression and providing information about the impact of treatments
- facilitate patient–clinician communication, thereby promoting shared decision making, leading to better meeting of patients' needs, improving patients' satisfaction and increasing their adherence to treatment
- monitoring outcomes to improve quality or to reward better care.

PROs can be used by clinicians as part of routine patient assessment and management, especially in longer-term conditions. They provide baseline information about patients' health-related quality of life to complement more traditional history taking and physiological measurement. Condition-specific PROs are used as one-time screening questionnaires – for example, in depression – with follow-up on patients triggered by scores above some predetermined threshold (Snyder and Aaronson, 2009). Measured again at subsequent visits, PROs can help evaluate disease progression or regression as well as the effects of treatment (Fung and Hays, 2008). It has also been argued that PROs can allow the identification of vulnerable patients and enable clinicians to undertake continuous assessment of quality of care (Valderas et al., 2008).

PROs information can be used to inform patients' decisions about the likely benefits of treatment, either as part of shared decision making or, more formally, as part of patients' decision tools. For example, Brundage et al. (2006) examined the effect on choice of treatment of providing patients with data on health-related quality of life from clinical trials. And, of course, as we have seen with Dr Tim Hughe's use of PROs in his consultations (p 29).

Feldman-Stewart and Brundage (2009) point to other, less obvious, benefits of PROs. They assert that their use by clinicians in monitoring health over time improves patients' memory of and ability to describe their problems. Also, PROs can highlight problems that patients experience, but might not have thought to raise them with their clinician if they were unaware of their relevance and which clinicians therefore assumed not to be of concern. Completion of a PRO instrument might in itself contribute to helping patients to feel cared for and the information provides a structured basis for patients' discussions with their clinician.

At the health system level, as in the NHS PROMs programme, cost constraints and the need for a reliable standard method of data collection permit only the minimum number of observations from patients to measure changes – one before a specific treatment and one after. In clinical use more frequent data collection might be more appropriate and informative. PRO data can be collected during each patient contact, or can be completed at home. Creative examples of the use of PROs – albeit in research settings – include use of the EQ-VAS in a daily patient diary, in order to monitor the impact on health-related quality of life of long-term changes and acute exacerbations experienced by patients with multiple sclerosis (Parkin *et al.*, 2004). The development of touch-screen computers and other electronic means of collecting PRO data offer potential for improving how PRO data are collected and used in clinical practice (Rose and Bezjak, 2009).

The availability of PROs to clinicians for use in their clinical practice has been enhanced by an initiative by the National Institutes of Health in the USA called the Patient Reported Outcomes Measurement Information System (PROMIS) (Broderick *et al.*, 2013). Although PROMIS is primarily intended to provide PROs that can be used as endpoints in clinical studies in research settings, it claims that it 'Provides data about the effect of therapy that cannot be found in traditional clinical measures' and Broderick *et al.* suggest that it might be used in routine practice, though they report being disappointed that there is little evidence of PROs in general being used in this way.

A review of the impact of the use of PROs in clinical practice (Marshall *et al.*, 2006) concluded that the feedback of patients' PRO data to clinicians had a significant impact on some processes of care – particularly on the diagnosis of mental health conditions – but that evidence on the impact on patient health status was inconsistent. Robust evaluation of the value of PROs in clinical practice is required – as indeed it is in all the uses of these data described here. The subsequent systematic review by Valderas *et al.* (2008) reported that most of the published studies that met their scientific criteria for inclusion found that using PROs had a positive impact on at least one aspect of the process outcomes assessed by study assessed. They concluded from this that 'there are some grounds for optimism in the possible impact of measurement of PRO in clinical practice (specifically in improving diagnosis and recognition of problems and patient–physician communication)'. However, they found that there is less good evidence about effects on patient health status, as these were less frequently assessed and also detected.

The effects on process therefore seem well-established, so much so that a study published in 2010 was entitled 'The use of patient reported outcomes becomes standard practice in the routine clinical care of lung–heart transplant patients' (Santana *et al.*, 2010). The authors based this claim on their finding that 'The routine clinical use of PROs measures in the clinic was well accepted by patients and clinicians and was associated with a reduction of the duration of visits.' Unfortunately, there was no assessment of whether the costs of using PROs matched the benefits, but it does suggest their potential effectiveness at a process level.

In order for PROs to be used in and be useful to clinical practice, such data must be acceptable to clinicians, and the instruments themselves must be seen as offering legitimate and relevant data. This makes the selection of the instruments to be used crucial – they must be supported by clear evidence of validity and reliability. PRO data must also be affordable and practical to collect – and not adversely affect the clinical workflow (Snyder and Aaronson, 2009).

There is clearly potential for PROs to confer benefit when used in the clinical context – but this depends on how the data are collected, how they are fed back to clinicians and how they are actually used by clinicians in consultations and monitoring. Unless clinicians actively use the data their patients provide, additional data collection is of little benefit.

Are PROs relevant to decisions about referral?

Snyder and Aaronson (2009) argue that one important factor in the usefulness of PROs in clinical practice is that there are clear links between PRO data and guidelines for practice and clinical pathways. This raises an interesting question: to what extent can and should PRO data play a role in referral guidelines and clinical judgements about treatment?

There are substantial variations in referral rates in the NHS (Clarke *et al.*, 2009). These variations have been noted as a cause for concern for many years, but addressing them presents considerable challenges. Reducing these differences in effect requires a change in the clinical decisions being made by individual referring GPs and there is a tension between the pursuit of consistency in treatment of patients across the NHS and clinical autonomy. Furthermore, as the NHS continues to place greater importance on responsiveness to patients and ensuring that patients' preferences are taken into account, this also presents a tension with attempts to introduce systematic approaches to demand management. These are aimed at improving the appropriateness of referrals but can also limit patients' choices.

The differences in referral rates are also mirrored in substantial differences in surgical intervention rates across the NHS. The explanation for these variations is unclear, suggesting that considerable idiosyncrasy in clinical decision making might exist at both primary and secondary care levels. A review of this issue concluded:

> Variations between GP practices' referral patterns and rates remain largely unexplained. Patient, practice and GP characteristics account for less than half of observed variation, the impact of social class is not clear-cut and 'no one variable or group of variables appears to be a predictor of variation'. There has been 'no relationship found between referral rates and age of GP, years of experience or membership of the [Royal College of General Practitioners]...', and there is 'conflicting evidence about the relationship between practice size and variation in referral rates'. (British Medical Association, 2009; phrases within quotes are taken from O'Donnell, 2000)

However, wider influences might affect the variation. For example, O'Donnell (2000) suggests that high levels of referrals are related to high levels of supply. Greater clinical consensus over what constitutes an appropriate referral and when treatment will benefit the patient could yield important benefits to overall patient health, improve how resources are used and potentially improve equity in access to care.

International use of PROs in referral management

How do other health systems address these issues? What can be learnt from how referrals and access to surgery are handled elsewhere? And is there any role for using PRO data to address this issue?

An example of how PRO-type instruments can be used in referral and treatment decisions is provided by the Canadian and New Zealand health care systems. Of course, there are important differences between these countries and England in terms of how health care is funded, provided and managed, which could limit the relevance of the experience there to the NHS. For example, an important context to the introduction of explicit patient prioritisation in both countries is that it was stimulated in part to address long waiting times (e.g. Noseworthy *et al.*, 2003). In contrast, England has addressed its waiting times problem largely by the use of waiting time targets; that is, using supply-side, rather than demand-side, initiatives.

With that caveat in mind, we now provide a brief summary of the points systems used in New Zealand and Canada, and the role of PROs in those systems, and then we consider the relevance of them to clinical decisions to refer and treat in the NHS.

For more than a decade, New Zealand has used a points system to determine patients' access to publicly funded elective surgery. Introduced in the mid-1990s (Hadorn and

Holmes, 1997a; 1997b), the aim is to develop standardised sets of explicit criteria that assess the extent to which patients have the ability to benefit from a range of elective surgical procedures. These criteria for assessing ability to benefit were applied consistently across the country, to ensure fairness in access to treatment for any given condition and also to facilitate direct comparisons of ability to benefit across different conditions and treatments.

Clinical Priority Assessment Criteria (CPAC) were developed and used in decisions about patient access to cataract surgery, coronary artery bypass graft, hip and knee replacement, cholecystectomy and tympanostomy tubes for otitis media with effusion. Patients with sufficient points under this system were guaranteed treatment within a short period through a surgical booking system. Those who do not have enough points to merit surgery, that is, they fall below an agreed clinical threshold, are not offered surgery. This is, in effect, an explicit form of rationing (Derrett, 2001).

An example of one aspect of the points system to prioritise patients for cataract surgery is one currently used in New Zealand's publicly funded health care system. There, an 'impact on daily living' questionnaire developed for self-completion by patients is used alongside the clinician's assessment about the improvement in health possible through treatment, as the basis for prioritising patients for cataract surgery. This approach is endorsed for use by the Royal Australian and New Zealand College of Ophthalmologists.

The principles underpinning this points system are summarised in Box 4.1, written by Dr Ray Naden and Alison Barber, who lead the management of elective surgery in the New Zealand Ministry of Health.

Box 4.1 Ethical principles underlying explicit prioritisation of patients for elective surgery

Dr Ray Naden[1] and Alison Barber[1]

The aim of points systems is to ensure horizontal equity in access to publicly-funded health care services, that is, patients with equal need and ability to benefit from treatments should have equal access to treatment, regardless of, for example, where they happen to live, their ethnicity, their education or income. Points systems work by providing an explicit and consistent basis for answering the following key questions.

Question 1: Is the treatment in the best interests of the patient? (i.e. is the patient's net ability to benefit, weighing up the benefits and the risks of treatment >0?)

Question 2: Is the treatment available to this patient? If everyone who needs it can have it, then no. Because taxpayer-funded health care budgets in New Zealand, as in the NHS, are limited, inevitably priorities for access to services must be made both overall (should more be spent on ophthalmology or on other areas of treatment and prevention?) and within any given clinical area (should more be spent on cataracts, or on other sorts of ophthalmological problems?).

Points systems are a means of making those judgements in a way that is fair, explicit and consistent. The use of points systems marks a departure from a reliance on paternalistic, potentially idiosyncratic, decisions by individual clinicians.

The points systems currently being used across elective surgical procedures in New Zealand entail a mix of PROs and clinical judgements. The points assigned to a given patient are based on two questions.

- What impact does the patient's condition have on his or her quality of life? This is clearly best judged by patients themselves. Existing PROs, such as the EQ-5D, are not always adequate for this, so bespoke PROs have been developed and validated for each area of elective surgery.
- To what extent is the patient's condition able to be ameliorated by treatment?

This is clearly best judged by clinicians – and the points system systematises these judgements.

The points system does use PROs, but as a complement to, rather than a substitute for, clinical judgements. Achieving clinical consensus about the way in which patients are assigned points is crucial to the success of the system.

The introduction of these points systems in New Zealand has conferred significant benefits.

- Important differences in access to surgery for people of equal need were revealed to exist by region, and were addressed.
- Important differences in access to surgery for people of equal need were revealed to exist by ethnicity, and were addressed.
- Important disparities between access to surgery within clinical areas (e.g. cataract surgery versus treatment for other ophthalmological conditions) were revealed and this has informed resource allocation decisions within that clinical area.
- Disparities between different areas of elective surgery, in terms of patients' relative ability to benefit, informs decisions about resource allocation between different clinical areas, affecting different groups of patients.

[1] New Zealand Ministry of Health

Similar schemes to these are also in use in Canada's social insurance system. For example, priority criteria are used to determine treatment for hip and knee replacement surgery (Arnett and Hadorn, 2003) and cataract surgery (Romanchuk et al., 2002).

Derrett (2005) noted the potential concern that the use of PROs in points systems might prompt patients to exaggerate their problems to game the system, but she found that, in practice, quantitative and qualitative analysis of the data suggested patient exaggeration was not an important influence on CPAC scores. Rather, she stated: 'The over-riding message from patients was of support for a 'fair' system in which patients in greater 'need' accessed surgery first – irrespective of whether or not they themselves were in the groups receiving surgery' (p. 36).

Arguably, one of the most important impacts of the points system has been on equity of access. One of the key aims of New Zealand's elective surgical reforms was to make the system fairer for patients and to ensure horizontal equity – that is, equal treatment for those with equal needs. Evidence on this has been reported from Counties Manukau, one of the poorest and most ethnically diverse regions of New Zealand. Historically, the Maori rate of elective surgery has been well below that in other ethnic groups of the population. As the points system was implemented, this gap has closed. The biggest changes were evident for hip and knee replacements, cardiac procedures and cataracts and, notably, the largest improvements in access occurred in the areas of greatest deprivation (Lindsay *et al.*, 2007). The implication is that assessing priority for treatment using explicit criteria that provide a consistent basis for referral and access to treatment can promote equity in access to health care.

However, the implementation and use of these points systems is not without its problems (Gauld and Derrett, 2000; Dew *et al.*, 2005; Derret *et al.*, 2013). Of critical importance is the validity of the specific PRO-type instruments that are used to award points: early versions of the CPAC scoring systems were not properly validated and were of questionable scientific merit as a means of judging patients' ability to benefit.

Furthermore, there is a fundamental challenge in developing scoring systems that are both sufficiently sensitive to facilitate judgements about relative ability to benefit within a given clinical area – such as ophthalmology – but also broad enough to facilitate legitimate comparisons of relative ability to benefit across different clinical areas.

PRO-based tools also give rise to the possibility of gaming behaviours by both patients and clinicians. In New Zealand, their introduction coincided with a period of reductions in real budgets, which posed particular challenges. Moreover, as Derret *et al.* (2013) have noted, context, funding and implementation issues such as '…periodic changes in central government policy, largely following high-profile negative incidents, as well as substantial capacity for regions to incrementally change the way in which they administer the system' can override the impact of such prioritisation approaches. And a Controller and Auditor's report in 2011 underlines the difficulties encountered with the prioritisation initiative, concluding that 'Despite the encouraging improvements made in the last 10 years, we do not yet have a system for scheduled services that can demonstrate national consistency and equitable treatment for all.' (Controller and Auditor General, 2011).

The potential role of points systems in the NHS

So what are the prospects for the use of these sorts of PRO-based tools in other health systems, such as the NHS? Might points-type systems be useful as a means of overcoming known variations in referral and treatment of patients? Does the PROs programme present an opportunity to capitalise on the pre-surgical collection of PROs, to facilitate explicit patient prioritisation?

The use of explicit patient prioritisation would mark a significant departure from current practice. Department of Health-sponsored research on referral guidelines has not promoted explicit scoring systems, but rather has focused on how to take patient preferences about treatment into account in the decision to refer (Clarke *et al.*, 2009).

On the other hand, Edwards *et al.* (2003) suggest that there is support among GPs, consultants, commissioners and patients in the NHS for a more explicit way of prioritising patients for treatment. Their results showed that all groups included in their survey agreed that the level of pain, rate of deterioration of the disease, level of distress and level of disability are factors that should have an influence on which patients receive treatment.

The key questions are whether the PROs now routinely collected in the NHS are sufficiently robust to be used in this way and whether they are adequate predictors of patients' ability to benefit from treatment.

The New Zealand points system does not use the EQ-5D, and a prospective study of the points system suggested that the EQ-5D is imperfect as a tool for predicting patient benefit (Derrett *et al.*, 2003). This suggests that purpose-built instruments may be required. Current work in New Zealand is focused on developing and validating, in partnership with both patients and clinicians, bespoke scoring tools. PROs are an important aspect of these, but are complementary to clinician judgements.

It therefore seems likely that the PRO data currently being collected in the NHS at baseline do not in themselves provide a sufficiently robust basis for referral guidelines. However, those data, combined with condition-specific data also being collected and combined with consensus clinical judgements, might be relevant. But as Derret *et al.* (2013) point out, developing and consistently implementing a points system is challenging, can have unintended consequences and highlights regional differences in service management and patient access.

PROs and other health professions

To date, most of the focus on PROs has been on doctors. This may reflect a belief that it is their performance that is most crucial in effecting improvement on patient-reported health from treatment. But what of the role of other health professionals? For example, the quantity and quality of nursing will have an effect on improvements in patient-reported health that is independent of doctors' quality.

Similarly, the services of allied health professionals may also be important to PROs. For example, the quantity and quality of physiotherapy is likely to exert an influence on improvement of patient-reported health following orthopaedic surgery (Devlin *et al.*, 2010). Barham and Devlin (2011) have emphasised the importance of nurses engaging with PRO data to improve nursing practices and clinical quality more generally.

The focus on doctors so far is probably due to the initial focus on surgical procedures, where the role of the clinician dominates and the need to get acceptance and support from powerful professional groups is most crucial. But, as PROs are rolled out across a wider range of NHS services, such as mental health, primary care and services for longer-term conditions, the quantity and quality of care, advice, supportive services and a wider range of health and social care services, is likely to become as − if not more − important in determining self-reported improvement in patients' health.

References

Appleby J, Devlin N (2004) *Measuring Success in the NHS. Using Patient-Assessed Health Outcomes to Manage the Performance of Health Care Providers*. London: King's Fund/ Dr Foster.

Arnett G, Hadorn DC (2003) Developing priority criteria for hip and knee replacement: results from the Western Canada Waiting List Project. *Canadian Journal of Surgery*, vol 46, no 4, pp 290–296.

Barham L, Devlin N (2011) Patient-reported outcome measures: implications for nursing. *Nursing Standard*, vol 25, no 18, pp 42–45.

British Medical Association (2009) *Factors Capable of Influencing an Increase in GP Referral Rates to Secondary Care (England only)*. London: British Medical Association Health Policy and Economic Research Unit. Available at: www.sheffield-lmc.org.uk/OG09/Factors%20 Caple%20of%20Influencing%20an%20increase%20in%20GP%20Referral%20Rates%20to%20 Secondary%20Care.pdf (accessed on 1 July 2015).

Broderick J, Morgan DeWitt E, Rothrock N, Crane P, Forrest C (2013) Advances in patient reported outcomes: The NIH PROMIS measure. *eGems* (Generating evidence and methods to improve patient outcomes), vol 1, issue 1, article 12. Available at: http://repository.academyhealth.org/cgi/ viewcontent.cgi?article=1015&context=egems (accessed 15 June, 2015).

Brundage M, Feldman-Stewart D, Leis A, Bezjak A, Pater JL (2006) Patients' judgments about the value of quality of life information when considering lung cancer treatment options. Abstracts of the 13th Annual Conference of the International Society for Quality of Life Research, Lisbon, Portugal, 10–14 October. *The QLR Journal*, suppl A-68, abstract no 1810.

Clarke A, Musila N, Le Maistre N, Black N, van der Meulen J (2009) *The REFER Project: Realistic effective facilitation of elective referral for elective surgical assessment*. Research report for the National Co-ordinating Centre for the National Institute for Health Research Service Delivery and Organisation Programme (NCCSDO). London: Royal College of Surgeons of England. Available at: www.netscc.ac.uk/hsdr/files/project/SDO_FR_08-1310-072_V01.pdf (accessed on 1 July 2015).

Controller and Auditor-General (2011) Progress in delivering publicly funded scheduled services to patients. Office of the Auditor General, Wellington. Available at: www.oag.govt.nz/2011/scheduled-services/docs/scheduled-services.pdf (accessed 15 June, 2015).

Derrett S (2001) Surgical prioritisation and rationing: some recent changes. *New Zealand Bioethics Journal*, vol 2, no 3, pp 3–6.

Derrett S (2005) *Booking Systems for Elective Services in New Zealand: Literature scan to identify any ethical issues of national significance*. A report to the National Ethics Advisory Committee. University of Keele, Staffordshire: Centre for Health Planning and Management. Available at: http://neac.health.govt.nz/system/files/documents/publications/bookingsystemselectiveservices.doc (accessed on 1 July 2015).

Derret S, Cousins K, Gauld R (2013) A messy reality: An analysis of New Zealand's elective surgery scoring system from media sources: 2000–2006. *International Journal of Health Planning and Management*, vol 28, no 1, pp 48–62.

Derrett S, Devlin N, Hansen P, Herbison P (2003) Prioritizing patients for elective surgery: A prospective study of clinical priority assessment criteria (CPAC) in New Zealand. *International Journal of Technology Assessment in Health Care*, vol 19, no 1, pp 91–105.

Devlin N, Parkin D, Browne J (2010) Patient Reported Outcome Measures in the NHS: new methods for analysing and reporting EQ-5D data *Health Economics*, vol 19, pp 886–905.

Dew K, Cumming J, McLeod D, Morgan S, McKinlay E, Dowell A, Love T (2005) Explicit rationing of elective services: implementing the New Zealand reforms. *Health Policy*, vol 74, no 1, pp 1–12.

Edwards RT, Boland A, Wilkinson C, Cohen D, Williams J (2003) Clinical and lay preferences for the explicit prioritisation of elective waiting lists: survey evidence from Wales. *Health Policy*, vol 63, no 3, pp 229–237.

Feldman-Stewart D, Brundage MD (2009) A conceptual framework for patient–provider communication: a tool in the PRO research toolbox. *Quality of Life Research*, vol 18, pp 109–114.

Fung C, Hays RD (2008) Prospects and challenges in using patient reported outcomes in clinical practice. *Quality of Life Research*, vol 17, no 10, pp 1297–302.

Gauld R, Derrett S (2000) Solving the surgical waiting list problem? New Zealand's booking system. *International Journal of Health, Planning and Management*, vol 15, no 4, pp 259–272.

Hadorn DC, Holmes AC (1997a) The New Zealand priority criteria project. Part 1: overview. *British Medical Journal*, vol 314, no 7074, pp 131–134.

Hadorn DC, Holmes AC (1997b) The New Zealand priority criteria project. Part 2: coronary artery bypass graft surgery. *British Medical Journal*, vol 314, no 7074, pp 135–138.

Lindsay G, Jackson G, Robinson T (2007) *Improving Access to Elective Surgery 1996/7 to 2005/6*. Report to Counties Manukau District Health Board.

Marshall S, Haywood K, Fitzpatrick R (2006) Impact of patient-reported outcome measures on routine clinical practice: a structured review. *Journal of Evaluation in Clinical Practice*, vol 12, no 5, pp 559–568.

NHS England (2014) Commissioning for quality and innovation (CQUIN): 2014/15 guidance February 2014. NHSE, London. Available at: www.england.nhs.uk/wp-content/uploads/2014/02/sc-cquin-guid.pdf (accessed 15 June, 2015).

Noseworthy TW, McGurran JJ, Hadorn DC (2003) Waiting for scheduled services in Canada: development of priority-setting scoring systems. *Journal of Evaluation in Clinical Practice*, vol 9, no 1, pp 23–31.

O'Donnell CA (2000) Variation in GP referral rates: what can we learn from the literature? *Family Practice*, vol 17, no 6, pp 462–71.

Parkin D, Rice N, Jacoby A, Doughty J (2004) Use of a visual analogue scale in a daily patient diary: modelling cross-sectional time-series data on health-related quality of life. *Social Science and Medicine*, vol 59, no 2, pp 351–360.

Romanchuk KG, Sanmugasunderam S, Hadorn DC; Steering Committee of the Western Canada Waiting List Project (2002) Developing cataract surgery priority criteria: results from the Western Canada Waiting List Project. *Canadian Journal of Ophthalmology*, vol 37, no 3, pp 145–154.

Rose M, Bezjak A (2009) Logistics of collecting patient reported outcomes (PROs) in clinical practice: an overview and practical examples. *Quality of Life Research*, vol 18, no 1, pp 125–136.

Santana M, Feeny D, Weinkauf J, Nador D, Kapasi A, Jackson K, Schafenacker M, Zuk D, and Lien D (2010) The use of patient reported outcomes becomes standard practice in the routine clinical care of lung–heart transplant patients. *Patient Relat Outcome Meas*. 2010 Jul, vol 1, pp 93–105.

Snyder CF, Aaronson NK (2009) Use of patient reported outcomes in clinical practice. *The Lancet*, vol 374, no 9687, pp 369–370.

Valderas JM, Alonso J, Guyatt GH (2008) Measuring patient reported outcomes: moving from clinical trials into clinical practice. *Medical Journal of Australia*, vol 189, no 2, pp 93–94.

CHAPTER 5

Hospitals: managing clinical quality

Clinical teams up and down the country are now measuring the quality of care that they provide to their patients, and all acute trusts are recording this information so that they can publish the first ever set of Quality Accounts alongside their financial Accounts for the year 2009/10. This will make the NHS the first health system in the world to systematically measure, record and openly publish the quality of care that it achieves. Our new approach to payments means that quality improvement is financially recognised and rewarded, making quality the watchword. (Professor the Lord Darzi in 'High quality care for all: Our journey so far', p. 4: Department of Health, 2009: Reproduced with permission under Crown Copyright.)

Lord Darzi rightly acclaims the English NHS as a global leader in the collection – via patient reported outcomes – of information directly bearing on quality of care. However, a central issue for Trusts is how such data can actually be used to improve performance, not just in terms of the quality of care provided to patients, but also in other dimensions such as the efficiency with which that care is delivered.

PRO data offer tremendous opportunities for providers to benchmark themselves against others and to monitor a key aspect of the quality of care that they deliver. This chapter examines how providers can use PRO data to facilitate dialogue between managers and clinicians and to identify actions that might be taken to improve quality and efficiency. It should be noted, however, that the NHS Health and Social Care Information Centre (HSCIC) reports PRO data not by hospital site, but by trust, as a result of the linkage arrangements with Hospital Episode Statistics (HES) and data quality problems with the reporting of site codes.

We begin by describing the PRO data that are currently available to providers in the English NHS, and how they are used within Quality Accounts (annual reports on the quality of services produced by every NHS trust: NHS Choices, 2015). We then look at ways in which PRO data can provide powerful analyses of issues of interest to health care providers and others who are concerned with how these organisations perform. Finally, we discuss the experience of Bupa, which led the world in pioneering the routine use of PRO data in the quality management of its (then) network of hospitals. The resulting knowledge base built up over more than a decade provides clear lessons for the NHS.

Using Patient Reported Outcomes to Improve Health Care,
First Edition. John Appleby, Nancy Devlin and David Parkin.
© 2016 John Wiley & Sons, Ltd. Published 2016 by John Wiley & Sons, Ltd.

What PRO data are available to NHS hospitals?

There are two ways in which data from the NHS PROMs programme are made available by the Health and Social Care Information Centre (HSCIC). Routine reports are published on the HSCIC website and patient-level data are available upon application, though of course with strict conditions for access and use.

Routine reporting currently (in the year 2015) has four elements. First, every month 'Key facts' for England as a whole are published, covering the current financial year to date and the previous financial year. These comprise the percentage of eligible patients who participate and, for each procedure and each PRO, the percentages of patients whose scores had improved, were unchanged or worsened. Second, there are monthly reports on data quality. Third, four times a year, data for each provider (NHS Trust or non-NHS provider) and commissioner (Clinical Commissioning Group (CCG – see later) of referring GP) are published as a spreadsheet, covering the same time periods. These data are labelled as provisional until they have been fully checked and analysed. The final version for each year, which includes additional analyses, is therefore generally published 2 years after the data are collected. These final reports are accompanied by a clickable map offering provider-level key facts. Fourth, there are special reports on topics such as more detailed analysis of the individual PROs and rates of complications.

Within the spreadsheets, it is possible to examine data for each provider and commissioner and to make comparisons with others and with England as a whole. One section covers 'Key facts', including rates of participation and, for each procedure and each PRO, the case-mix adjusted average health gain, measured by the change in scores derived from pre-surgery and post-surgery questionnaires. These are automatically compared with the national averages and are presented as actual figures and as charts. Another section offers a comparison of the same data for up to 10 providers or commissioners. A third section provides, for each procedure and each PRO, funnel plots (described in Chapter 2) covering all providers or commissioners, with the ability to highlight a particular provider or commissioner.

An important feature of the patient-level PRO data is that they can be linked with other routine NHS data sets, for example, Hospital Episode Statistics (HES – patient-level data compiled from individual patient hospital records) and, for hip and knee procedures, the National Joint Register (NJR) database. The linkage of PROs to HES hugely increases the value of the information and has permitted much more in-depth exploration of, for example, possible reasons for variations in health-related quality of life outcomes between trusts. Some examples of this work are detailed next.

Quality Accounts

A key outlet for PRO data are NHS Trusts' Quality Accounts, which must be produced by any organisation that provides services under an NHS standard contract, has over 50 staff and a turnover greater than £130 000 per annum, including non-NHS bodies. They are required to report and comment on PRO data for any of the elective procedures that they provide. These have to be shared with local commissioners – CCGs and NHS England Area Teams – and scrutineers – Health Watch and Health and Well-being Boards. They are then published via the NHS Choices website.

Requirements for presentation include reporting a comparison of the Trust's PROs scores with the national averages and with those NHS Trusts and NHS Foundation Trusts with the highest and lowest scores, for at least two reporting periods. The Trust must also give reasons why their PRO scores are at the level that they are, and state what actions they have taken, are taking or intend to take to improve their scores and thereby the quality of its services. Box 5.1 gives an example of the PROs content of Quality Accounts for one provider.

Box 5.1 PROs in Quality Accounts: an example

North Middlesex University Hospital NHS Trust comprises a large general hospital in North London and two smaller community hospitals. It was rated in 2014 by the Care Quality Commission as 'Requires Improvement'. The Trust's Quality Accounts for 2013–2014 start by outlining their quality improvement priorities for the year. This includes initiating a clinical audit and effectiveness strategy for 2014–2017 with the aims of 'evidence-based best practice, governance and monitoring and clinical outcome and benchmarking'. Their first priority within this relates to compliance with the NHS elective surgery PROMs programme. The proportion of patients completing the PROs questionnaires is overall 87.9% of those eligible, which the Trust says is low and is particularly low for hip surgery.

The Trust proposes to set up a system for identifying patients who have groin hernia surgery, knee replacements and hip replacements (the Trust does not perform varicose vein repairs) and ensuring that patients are properly informed about the questionnaires and understand the importance of completing them. A target is set to increase compliance with PROMs to above 95%. The actual actions are to set up a database which identifies who should be completing the questionnaires; ensure that the data are discussed at specialty meetings and the clinical business unit risk and quality meeting; and make the data part of the key performance indicators discussed bi-monthly at the Trust's' clinical effectiveness group.

The Trust then reports for each of the three operations covered by the PROMs programme data from April 2013–September 2013 and April 2012–March 2013. It reports the scores for each PROM in each period for the Trust, the national average and the lowest and highest scores nationally. It comments on the data for each surgical intervention, for example concerning groin hernia surgery that:

> The data is consistent with the hospital's own internal monitoring and reporting of performance against this indicator. The Trust's performance has usually been broadly in line with the national average for this measure over time with slight improvement seen between the reporting periods shown above.

It states for all three interventions that the actions that it will take to improve its PRO scores are 'Ensuring that PROMs becomes a key clinical effectiveness target for the trust to concentrate on during 2014/15 … demonstrated by improvements in both coverage rates (the number of patients surveyed) and positive outcomes.'

The impact of the PROMs programme on the Trust therefore appears at this stage to be reassurance that the data have not demonstrated any serious problems with any of the surgical interventions covered by PROs, but a recognition that the data themselves need to be improved. This leads them to suggest improvements to administrative processes rather than clinical issues, but there is a presumption that improved data and making it more visible to clinical teams may have the effect of improving care and therefore outcomes.

The responses of the Trust to their PRO data suggest that the emphasis is on the aim of the Quality Accounts to provide and reinforce a focus on quality and quality improvement by providers. This includes the ability to benchmark performance and to promote improvements in care. However, an aim is also to improve transparency by providing commissioners and the public with information on the quality of care provided by their local health care services so as to improve local accountability and choice. The presentation of data specified by NHS England seems much better suited to the first set of aims than the second, in particular informing the general public, whose understanding of what PROs scores mean may be limited at best.

Understanding outcome variations

Variations in levels of service and outcomes are one of the certainties of health and health care in every country and type of health care system – see, for example, Box 5.2 which discusses Sweden's experience of PROs. It is therefore no surprise that PRO data reveal variations in the health of patients and in the improvements that they experience as a result of treatment; between hospitals, between clinicians in hospitals and between patients with different characteristics. This will rightly lead to questions about why some hospitals and clinicians appear to perform better or worse than others and why some patients report more or less benefit than others. Understanding the reasons associated with good and poor outcomes will be important.

Box 5.2 PROs in Sweden: national quality registers and population surveys

Evalill Nilsson[1] and Kristina Burström[2]

Sweden's 21 Region and County Councils that run health services increasingly encourage the evaluation of health care from the patients' perspective, using patient-reported outcome measures. Councils also use such measures to monitor the health of the population across regions and counties.

Stockholm County Council, for example, has used the EQ-5D in population health surveys since 1998. These surveys, sent to representative samples of 50 000 people, obtain a response rate of nearly two thirds using a cross-sectional design. Results have been presented by age, sex, socioeconomic groups and disease groups (Burström, 2001). The large sample size allows comparisons between local areas. Results were presented for each of the 39 districts and municipalities in the county and as an aggregate of the 16 socially disadvantaged residential areas that have been part of a special effort to improve living conditions for those living in the most deprived areas ('Storstadssatsningen'). Reports have been published which compared area differentials in social determinants of health (e.g. trust in others, smoking, alcohol, physical inactivity and eating habits) and PRO measures such as EQ-5D dimensions and EQ VAS scores (Burström, 2014). The results were age-standardised, stratified by sex and short and long education.

Results generally showed a social gradient in patient reported outcomes at the area level: in other words, the more disadvantaged area, the worse health-related quality of life, with some exceptions. The area gradient for women in reported problems in the anxiety/depression component of the EQ-5D measure is shown in Figure 5.1. The gradient in the mean VAS score among women is shown in Figure 5.2.

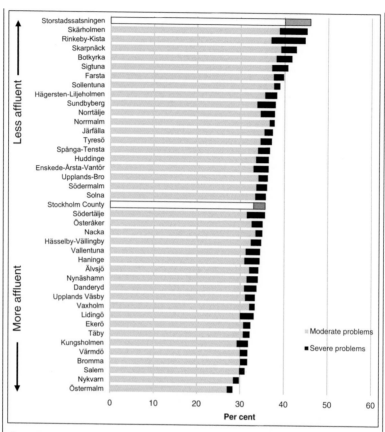

Figure 5.1 Proportion (%) with moderate and severe problems in the EQ-5D dimension anxiety/depression, by areas in Stockholm, Sweden, women 18–84 years. Source: Burström *et al.* (2014) reproduced with permission.

These data have been used by public health officials on a local level and have been put forward as a good example of how to utilise and display results to policy makers. The EQ-5D has also been included in face-to-face interviews among homeless people in Stockholm as an attempt to cover hard-to-reach groups in the assessment of population health (Sun, 2012). The considerable group and area differentials in health-related quality of life, living conditions and health-related behaviours and in life expectancy may contribute to further in-depth discussion among policy-makers on relevant actions to take to improve health and reduce inequalities in health between groups and areas.

The most systematic use of patient-reported data in the Swedish health care system today is seen in the National Quality Registers (NQRs). These list individualised data regarding patient problems, medical interventions and outcome after treatment. The registers are designed to be used in an integrated and active way for continuous

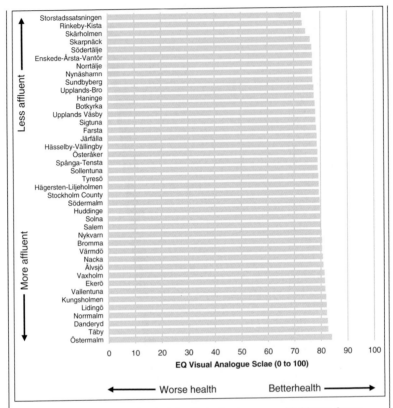

Figure 5.2 Mean EQ VAS score by area in Stockholm, Sweden, women, 18–84 years. Source: Burström *et al.* (2014) reproduced with permission.

learning, improvement, research and management to create the best possible health and care, together with the individual patients.

The NQRs are annually monitored and are certified at three levels. To reach the second level a register now must incorporate patient reported outcomes, and special governmental NQR funding is designated to support this development as part of an ambitious drive from the Ministry of Health and Social Affairs to increase use of patient-reported outcome data as a means for quality improvement work in the Swedish health care system.

A review of the annual applications for financial support for 2015 has shown that almost all registers report including some patient-reported measure, either to measure outcomes in terms of health-related quality of life, symptoms and functional ability (PROM), or to measure patient satisfaction (PREM, patient-reported experience measures), or both.

Figure 5.3 summarises the scope of PRO and PRE measures currently included in registers. The single most used measure was the EQ-5D.

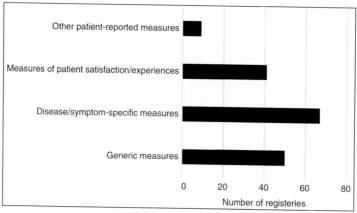

Figure 5.3 Overview of the current self-reported inclusion of PROMs and PREMs in the Swedish National Quality Registers. Source: Burström *et al.* (2014). NB: The most common generic measure was the EQ-5D (around 35 registers) and the SF-36/RAND-36 (around 10 registers). Of the 10% or so reporting not having any PRO or PRE measures in the register, most reported planning for inclusion in the near future. Further, several of the registers already using these measures reported planning for an extended use. NB: 'Other patient-reported measures' included measures of work situation, lifestyle factors, and burden of care from the perspectives of the relatives of the patient. (From the 108 annual applications for funding for 2015)

Twenty registers presented examples of how patient-reported data from the register had been used in quality improvement work. Examples included use for shared decision making in clinical encounters (most common), as a basis for care plans, clinical decision aids and patient overviews, and treatment guidelines, as indications for surgery (patient and professional assessments may be incongruent), to monitor complications after the patient has left the hospital (especially important regarding the increasing amount of ambulatory care), and to improve patient information (Nilsson *et al.*, 2015).

An example of the use of this data in shared decision making is the new *Visual and Analysis Platform* (VAP) of the National Swedish MS (Multiple Sclerosis) Register. The current integrated medical and patient-reported results (including EQ-5D data) of a selected patient in comparison to a matching reference group estimated on the basis of data from the register is visualised in real-time in pedagogical, easy-to-interpret spider diagrams, to aid in further clinical management decisions and shared decision making.

Nine NQRs were found to have published scientific articles about the benefits of using patient-reported data; among them, the Swedish Hip Arthroplasty Register – which has used EQ-5D data to compare health outcomes between providers, to explore surgical and patient-related determinants of outcomes and to stimulate clinical improvement work (Rolfson *et al.*, 2011).

[1] The Research & Development Department of Local Health Care, Region Östergötland, Sweden

[2] Karolinska Institutet, Department of Learning, Informatics, Management and Ethics, Health Outcomes and Economic Evaluation Research Group & Karolinska Institutet, Department of Public Health Sciences, Equity and Health Policy Research Group & Stockholm County Council, Health Care Services

The issue of case mix

When comparing different providers' PRO scores, it is important to account for factors that affect outcomes but are not due to variations in the quality of care. For example, the average age of patients treated may differ between different providers and that may affect the outcomes that can be achieved, irrespective of how effective their care is. Scores are therefore adjusted to take account of the mix of cases seen by providers. Box 5.3 shows how the NHS does this for its PROMs programme.

Box 5.3 The NHS case-mix adjustment method

The NHS case-mix adjustment method has two stages. First, regression analysis is used to calculate the average impact of case-mix variables on PRO scores over all patients. This is used to estimate for each provider the average PRO score that would be expected for its particular mix of those variables. How much its expected and actual outcomes differ is a measure of its performance.

However, this only gives a comparison with a hypothetical provider that has the same case mix, rather than with other real providers. The second stage is therefore to recalculate each provider's outcomes so that they can be compared to a standardised case mix. This mix is the average level of the case-mix variables over all providers, which by definition also generates the all-providers average PRO score.

This method, known as indirect standardisation, is illustrated by Figure 5.4. This shows a very simple adjustment to the post-surgery PROs score (Q2) using one case-mix variable, the pre-surgery PRO score (Q1). The regression line shows that at all levels of Q1 there is on average an improvement following surgery (the line lies above the Q1 = Q2 line, meaning no change in health); Q2 is higher with higher Q1; but the size of the improvement (the difference between Q2 and Q1) is smaller with higher Q1.

For provider A, its average post-surgery score is Q2a and the change in PROs score unadjusted for case mix is $\Delta Q = Q2a-Q1a$. Its expected score is Q2b and it therefore has performed better than expected. Performance can be quantified as Q2a-Q2b; if this is positive, the provider achieves on average results greater than those predicted; negative if worse than predicted; and zero if as predicted. This difference is applied to the all-provider Q2 score, which is Q2d, to give the estimated actual score for Provider A if it had the all-provider case mix. This score, Q2c, is calculated so that $Q2c - Q2d = Q2a - Q2b$, which means $Q2c = Q2d + (Q2a - Q2b)$. The relevant Q1 comparator for this is the all-provider Q1 score, so the case-mix adjusted change in PROMs score for Provider A is $\Delta Q' = Q2c - Q1$.

This explanation is adapted from Nuttall *et al.* (2013). Full details of the method are given in Department of Health (2012) and NHS England Analytical Team (2013).

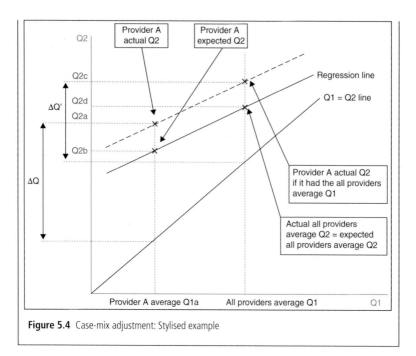

Figure 5.4 Case-mix adjustment: Stylised example

Accounting for case mix permits a fairer comparison of the provision of care within a hospital, but it does not fully cover the issue of a hospital's performance as measured by outcomes since case mix is to some extent under the control of the hospital. For example, it is reasonable in looking at improvements in health achieved to take account of the average severity of patients on admittance. If the hospital simply takes all who could be treated, this is a factor beyond its control. However, severity on admission may to some extent be determined by treatment thresholds decided within the hospital, and by policies concerning referrals to outpatients by GPs. Examining PRO data on pre-treatment health status gives an insight into this issue. Variations between different hospitals have consequences for equity of access for patients, capacity or opportunity to benefit from treatment and also for the efficient use of resources.

Examining variations in health and health care using PROs
In looking at the issue of variations, linkage between PROs and HES data provides access to many variables that are relevant to analyses, in particular a very rich set of patient characteristics. Researchers at the London School of Hygiene and Tropical Medicine have undertaken analyses around variations that not only illuminate important issues directly, but also demonstrate the power of PRO data to do that. The four studies described next examine variations between hospitals, consultant teams, different patient groups and the public and private sector.

The thresholds issue might lead to a suggestion that the more surgery a hospital does, the lower the average levels of need amongst treated patients will be and as a result less benefit generated per patient. Black *et al.* (20142014) published evidence using PRO data that this has not been an important factor. With an increase in surgery rates, there have been very small declines in the pre-operative PRO score for knee replacements and varicose vein repairs and a slight reduction in health gain measured by the disease-specific PRO score for varicose vein repairs, but otherwise no changes have been detected. The authors conclude that commissioners cannot justify policies to reduce surgical rates on the grounds of avoiding inappropriate operations or increasing cost-effectiveness.

Because PRO data are available at the level of consultant team, it is possible to examine variations between them. Varagunam *et al.* (2014) have argued that PROs might be better for comparing consultant surgeons' outcomes using hip and knee replacement and hernia repair than mortality. The evidence that they presented was that PROs are far more sensitive to differences between consultant teams, in particular in detecting relatively very poor outcomes.

Differences between how and when individual patients are treated are clearly important if Trusts are to make decisions in line with the equity goals of the NHS. Neuburger *et al.* (2012) examined differences in the severity and duration of disease amongst hip and knee replacement patients according to their sociodemographic characteristics. Using the Oxford Hip Score and the Oxford Knee Score, their study showed that women had more severe pain and disability than men on average but less often had longstanding problems; that average severity amongst South Asian and black patients was higher than in white patients and moreover black patients had longstanding problems; and patients from deprived areas had more severe disease. It is suggested that this is because non-white and deprived patients often have hip and knee replacement surgery later in the course of their disease.

An important and controversial policy issue is the use of private sector providers for NHS patients, and their relative performance in improving health is a key element of that. Chard *et al.* (2011) compared PROs in independent sector treatment centres (ISTCs) and NHS providers. The case mix of patients differed between them, though the differences were small; ISTC patients were healthier, had less severe pre-operative symptoms and were more affluent. NHS providers' patients undergoing joint replacements had poorer outcomes and reported complications more often, but there were no significant differences in outcomes for hernia or varicose veins, except that NHS patients more often reported poor results after hernia repair and additional surgery after varicose vein surgery. Again, these differences were small (see Box 5.4).

Box 5.4 Public or private? Does it matter to health outcomes who owns the means of production?

A controversial issue for the English NHS has been the use by the NHS of non-NHS health care providers. The separation of commissioning and the provision of care in the English NHS — changes that stretch back to reforms implemented in the early 1990s — have allowed state commissioners to purchase secondary care on behalf of their residents not just from NHS hospitals but independent sector providers too. More recently, patients have had the option of choosing non-NHS providers with their care paid for by the NHS.

While there may be objections to the use of the independent sector in this way, arguably what matters to patients and commissioners of care is whether there are systematic differences in the quality of care between state and independent sector providers.
PROMs data collected from NHS patients treated in both sectors provides some insight
into this issue.

A simple comparison between both sectors suggests a mixed picture. As Figure 5.5
shows, based on 1 year's PROMs data (2013–2014), the percentage of patients reporting an improvement in their health related quality of life (as measured by changes in
the EQ-5D index) for those treated by the independent sector was slightly higher than
those treated by NHS hospitals for hip and knee replacements, but slightly lower or
those undergoing hernia repair operations.

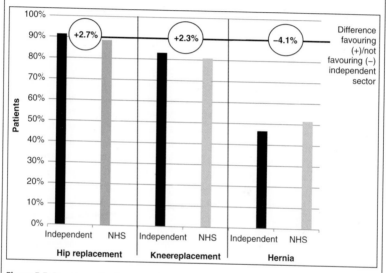

Figure 5.5 Percentage of patients treated in NHS or independent hospitals reporting an improvement
in health related quality of life. Source: Data: HSCIC (2014)

Other, more sophisticated and comprehensive studies have found similar results.
For example, Chard *et al.* (2011) found that patients treated by the independent
sector (but paid for by the NHS) tended to be healthier with slightly less severe
conditions than those treated by the NHS. While they found that PROs for hip and
knee replacement were slightly poorer for patients treated in NHS hospitals, differences were less clear cut for hernia and varicose vein patients. Gutacker *et al.*
(2013b) found similar results more indirectly based on a tendency for hospitals
with higher proportions of elective work to obtain better health outcomes coupled
with the fact that independent hospitals tend to carry out far less emergency
activity.

Average scores for hospitals will hide the variation within hospitals and between patients. Consequently, part of the variation in average PRO scores may, in some cases, be due to outlier scores for some patients. Equally, similar average scores can conceal very different distributions of scores between hospitals.

Comparative analysis of the individual questions that comprise the PRO scores will also be relevant as responses to these questions are also likely to vary. In addition, patterns of responses or changes post-operatively, particularly health-related aspects of patients' lives (e.g. pain, mobility and anxiety) might indicate where effort is needed to improve overall PRO results.

How do provider characteristics affect outcomes measured by PROs?

If there is one question providers need to ask themselves, which in any case will be asked of them, it is this: what is it about the nature of the hospital and the care provided that gives rise to the outcomes reported by patients?

There is considerable research literature investigating the reasons for variations in hospital performance on a whole variety of measures – from lengths of stay to infection rates and mortality. There will be similar research seeking to explain variations in PRO results in terms of the characteristics of hospitals, for example their size and type; inputs to care measured by, for example, staff to patient ratios; workload, capacity and the volume of activity and other factors related to providers, including measures concerned with primary care.

What such research will reveal about the explanations for any observed variation in PROs is an empirical matter. However, analogous research into the causes of variations in hospital mortality has suggested that a significant proportion of the variation can be explained by hospital and primary care factors. For example, a high proportion of all admissions being emergencies and a low number of hospital and primary care doctors per bed and per head of population, respectively, are all associated with higher in-hospital mortality (Jarman *et al.*, 1999). It would be surprising if similar associations were not found in the case of PROs – if not exactly the same factors or strength of association.

Providers should draw on the results of PRO variation research as it emerges to inform their strategies for improving their PRO performance. In the meantime, evidence of poor performance relative to other hospitals, as revealed by the data published in Quality Accounts, should prompt internal action to explore the data in detail so as to assess its significance. The evidence can then be reviewed with the clinical teams in order to identify possible explanations for the PROs results, and make changes to improve care.

Incentives

In the English NHS, providers face a number of system reform incentives designed to improve their performance, from patient choice to the fixed price tariff of Payment by Results. It is arguable, however, that the actual impact of such levers on the quality of care has been at best attenuated, as a result of the dearth of information on quality that is available for patients to use in making their choices, and the nature of the tariff which, again due to the relative lack of data on quality, acts, potentially at least, mainly on costs, regardless of the possible impact on quality.

Accepting PROs as a key measure of quality has, as noted in Chapter 3, the power to strengthen the influence that choice can have over providers' quality of care and, through mechanisms such as Commissioning for Quality and Innovation (CQUIN) (see Chapter 6), the ability to connect payments directly with outcomes.

Although PROs have the potential to strengthen system reform incentives such as choice and Payment by Results, these operate at the level of providers as organisations. However, just as budgetary devolution through, for example, Service Line Management (Foot *et al.*, 2012), more closely aligns the responsibility within a provider between the individuals and teams directly involved in decisions to commit resources and actual budgets, so the reporting of PROs as part of the SLM process can add the link between inputs and outcomes in a way that provides incentives that not only act on the professionalism of staff, but also possibly on their (or, more likely, team/specialty) financial interests.

Linking performance to pay, or, more commonly, to access to resources for a department or specialty, are not new, of course (and neither are they without some contention). However, PROs may well offer an advantage over other attempts to internalise external incentives, such as waiting time targets, as they are more directly concerned with clinical interests and motivation – the quality of care as it impacts on patient health.

PROs, costs and hospital efficiency

An important issue for providers is the measurement and monitoring of productivity and efficiency. What is the relationship between costs, the clinical quality of the care provided, and patient reported outcomes? And is there scope for improving efficiency?

Hospital managers probably have a very good understanding of how their input use relates to the production of services: they know which levers to pull to produce more activity and how the production of those services relates to cost. However, given that the collection and publication of PRO data is still at an early stage, managers probably have a less clear understanding of which levers to pull to improve patient health. The use of PRO-based performance indicators and the likelihood of revenue being linked to that performance, either indirectly (via patient choice and Payment by Results) or directly (via CQUIN payments), should create stronger pressures for managers to understand not just how their hospital's performance compares with others – but also the causes of any differences.

What the data will inevitably show is that performance and efficiency varies between hospitals. What will also be inevitable, as noted previously, will be the need for providers to analyse the underlying reasons for such variation. Poor performance will be due to a number of reasons. For example, outcomes might be good, but produced at high cost, or costs might be low, but outcomes poor.

Analyses using the NHS PRO data have already illuminated some of these issues. Box 5.5 gives details of some studies that have been published on different aspects of the efficiency with which hospitals generate improvements in health as measured by changes in PRO scores. Again, they also demonstrate the potential of PRO data and we can expect many more studies examining key aspects of efficiency, leading to better and more cost-effective care.

Box 5.5 Analysing efficiency in how hospitals produce health

The NHS PROMs programme facilitates a fundamental rethink about what hospital efficiency means and how it is measured. Most analyses of hospital production and cost functions, leading to estimates of efficiency, have examined variations between hospitals in the production of health *care* as the output of interest. PRO data enable a redefinition of output to focus on *health*. Hospital efficiency can then be measured by the extent to which hospitals achieve improvements in patient health given their inputs, resource use and other relevant factors, relating to both service delivery and the patients themselves.

Analyses of hospital performance start by identifying variations between hospitals and then try to understand which factors are associated with either very good or very poor performance. An important element is whether or not these factors are under the control of the hospital, or are 'environmental'. But variations in output do not, on their own, demonstrate variations in efficiency; that is, how the production of health relates to the hospital's use of inputs. These approaches, deriving from production economics, have been widely used to analyse and explain the differences between hospitals' efficiency in the production of services. The same analyses using PRO data facilitate, for the first time, analyses of the relative efficiency of providers in producing health.

One of the key debates about costs and quality has been whether improving quality is expensive, thereby justifying the higher costs that some providers have, or alternatively that improved quality leads to lower cost by, for example, reducing re-admissions. It has also been suggested that both of these might apply, depending on the context. When quality is poor, initiatives that improve quality also lower costs, but at some point extra quality requires extra expenditure. Gutacker et al. (2013a) analysed cost and PRO data for providers and found weak evidence in favour of this relationship for hip replacement surgery, but in general found little or no relationship between costs and PROMs outcomes. This is an interesting finding that needs to be explored at a less aggregate level than comparing aggregate data from all providers.

Another way to view the link between costs and PROs is to examine cost-effectiveness, as discussed in Chapter 7 along with the measurement of the productivity of the NHS in aggregate.

Looking at PROs scores tells us that providers vary in how much their patients' health overall health is improved, but what does that mean in terms that are recognisable to patients, clinicians and the general public? Gutacker et al. (2013b) employed the true richness of the PRO data by analysing differences between providers in improvements in the different dimensions of the EQ-5D for hip replacement patients. They found that the greatest variability was in how much providers improved patients' mobility and their ability to carry out their usual activities, rather than reducing pain and discomfort, alleviating anxiety and depression and enabling better self-care. This may suggest which aspects of clinical care providers ought to examine to improve quality. However, the authors also pointed out that in calculating overall PROs scores mobility and usual activities have a relatively low weight, so that these scores may give a partial and even perhaps misleading account of differences in provider performance.

What can the NHS learn from the independent health care sector?

Bupa Hospitals first started routine collection of patient-reported outcome data in 1998, prompted by the case of the rogue gynaecologist Rodney Ledward. Ledward practised in the NHS as well as for Bupa in the private sector. Following revelations of Ledward's gross malpractice, Bupa's then Medical Director, Andrew Vallance-Owen, reviewed activity and other performance statistics for Ledward but found that there were no '…deaths, no readmissions, no complaints – there was nothing to tell us about him. There were patients who clearly had serious complications but we knew nothing about it. It made me determined to collect patient reported outcomes' (Coombes, 2008, p. 1465).

Over the past decade, Bupa Hospitals (now Spire Health care) collected PRO data on more than 100 000 patient episodes. Although initially data collection covered a wide range of procedures, now the focus is on one or two sentinel procedures for each specialty, using generic measures, such as the SF-36, and condition-specific questionnaires, such as the VF-14 and the Oxford Hip and Knee Scores.

While the original stimulus for collecting PROs lay in a desire to spot clinical bad apples, it was clear that PROs offered the potential for continuous quality improvement and to provide feedback to GPs and patients. Moreover, with the PROs results (at hospital level) posted on their websites, Bupa Hospitals were able to promote and market the health-related quality of life benefits of the interventions they provided.

Feedback to health professionals developed over time, with straightforward bar charts of before and after results being supplemented with statistical control Shewhart charts detailing results relative to the mean for individual consultants together with limits set at +/– 3 standard deviations to indicate exceptional outliers (see Vallance-Owen et al. 2004).

For Dr Vallance-Owen, the argument in favour of collecting and using PRO data is clear:

> How can we know if a process brings benefits and continues to improve it without measuring the outcome, and how can we rely on process alone when the evidence shows such widespread variation and inconsistency in process in clinical practice? For patients, there is much more to success than alive or dead. How often have we heard: 'They said my hip replacement went well, but I am now housebound' or 'He says I have a good flow rate in my bypass graft, but I still get pain at 10 metres?' (Vallance-Owen, 2008, p 344)

The collection and analysis of PROs enabled Bupa to change clinical practices in its hospitals. For example, in one case, low scores prompted a hospital to change its care pathway for hysterectomy; in another, it identified a need to communicate more realism to patients concerning their expectations about the outcome of treatment. Further details of how Bupa implemented its use of PROs, and the benefits this yielded, are given in Box 5.5. In New Zealand too, the county's largest not-for-profit health insurers, Southern Cross Health Society, is just embarking on an on-line collection system for patient reported outcome measures (see Box 5.6).

Box 5.5 PROs in the independent health care sector

Andrew Vallance-Owen[1]

We started developing the routine measurement of PROs in Bupa's hospitals in 1997/8 following an incident from which it became clear that we had little idea of what happened to patients after their discharge from hospital, that is, what health benefit (or not) had been gained from their treatment.

We researched health status surveys and decided to use the Short Form 36 (SF-36). Patients were asked to complete the survey before their surgery, then again 3 months later to get a measure of health gain. Initially we also tried 6 weeks and 6 months but found the most useful data and best response rates at 3 months. After a successful pilot in a small number of hospitals, the programme was extended to all 25 Bupa Hospitals in the UK, offering the survey to all patients having common operations and eventually gaining 70–80% response rates overall.

The programme was started to give assurance that our patients were generally benefitting from their treatment, but it soon became apparent that feeding back PRO data to hospitals and consultants was a driver for quality improvement and that putting the PROMs data on hospital websites helped patients (usually advised by their GPs) to make more informed decisions about which providers they wanted to go to.

Bupa's work on the routine collection of PROMs became known in the wider health care system, but it was not until the Department of Health commissioned a significant academic study from the London School of Hygiene and Tropical Medicine in 2007 (Browne et al., 2007), that moves began to develop the NHS PROMs Programme.

Private Healthcare Information Network (PHIN)

PHIN developed from an initiative started by the UK's private hospitals called the Hellenic Project. This project was about building a common approach to the collection and analysis of clinical and other data across all the UK's independent hospitals; membership was voluntary but most hospitals became involved.

PHIN, an independent company limited by guarantee (not-for-profit), was established in July 2012. It receives data from its member organisations, taken from administrative and billing systems, clinical reporting and submissions to the NHS and regulators. Working closely with its members, the NHS and other partners, PHIN uses this data to create information designed to be as useful as possible to patients. Currently, it is publishing information covering approximately 200 hospitals and over 1 million patient admissions each year. Working with its members, PHIN started developing a potential PROMs programme in 2013.

Competition and Markets Authority (CMA)

In April 2012 the CMA started an investigation into the supply or acquisition of private health care in the UK; this focused principally on private hospitals and consultants working in private practice. The Final Order was published in October 2014 (CMA, 2014) and, amongst other things, mandates all operators of private health care facilities in the UK (and their consultants) to provide private patient episode data for processing and publication by the information organisation. PHIN has been confirmed as the 'information organisation'.

The types of data to be collected and published by PHIN are laid down in the Order; these include agreed measures of patient feedback and/or satisfaction and procedure-specific measures of improvement in health outcomes. These requirements fit well with the programme PHIN has been developing in conjunction with private providers and there is already a consensus building on around eight PROMs that could consistently be applied in appropriate hospitals across the sector.

The routine collection of PROMs was initiated in the independent sector and that work will now be continuing under the auspices of PHIN where the hope is that comparative data on up to eight PROMs may be published within the next 2 years.

---

¹Chair, Private Healthcare Information Network.

Box 5.6 PROs in New Zealand: online data collection
Sarah Gardner[1]

As part of its work to improve quality for patients, New Zealand's largest health insurer Southern Cross Health Society (a not-for-profit Friendly Society) is piloting the collection of PRO data. Getting the best value care for its members means funding quality health care at cost-effective prices and a crucial part of this is the patient's perspective.

Collection of patient reported outcome measures began in 2015 and will provide valuable data alongside existing surveys monitoring patients' experience of care which collects qualitative data about practitioners and facilities. While analysed separately, the two complement each other and will provide a holistic view of the patients' experience of clinical care and outcomes from their surgery.

The PROMs pilot will cover a wide range of surgery including:
- hip and knee replacements
- carpal tunnel
- cataracts
- prostate
- hysterectomy
- cardiac.

These surgeries represent around half of the overall surgery volume funded by Southern Cross Health Society.

The pilot will use the online version of the EQ-5D–5L instrument, which will be emailed to Society members pre-operatively as part of the consent process for surgery. Participating members will then be tracked through the claims system to enable a follow-up survey to be issued within an appropriate timeframe post-operatively.

Implementing the online version of EQ-5D–5L relies on getting the electronic survey to members at an appropriate point, relative to their scheduled date of surgery, type of procedure and subsequent recovery timeframe. Clear criteria and systems for gathering data have been developed to ensure the survey reaches members at the right time and maximises response rates. This includes different time frames for the post-operative follow-up survey depending on the procedure.

In order to thoroughly test the system by which member information is captured and use of the electronic version of EQ-5D-5L, the PROMs pilot will initially use the generic EQ-5D–5L tool without condition-specific measures linked to each procedure. It is likely that condition-specific PROMs will be built into the second phase of this work.

Clinicians have expressed an interest in viewing the PROMs results, particularly when benchmarked anonymously against peers. It is hoped that by sharing the data with providers, the Society can foster an environment where clinicians can learn from the findings, enhancing both the process of quality assurance and leading to continuous quality improvement.

[1] Southern Cross Health Society

References

Black N, Varagunam M, Hutchings A. (2014) Influence of surgical rate on patients' reported clinical need and outcomes in English NHS. *J Public Health* (2014) vol 36, no 3, 497–503. doi: 10.1093/pubmed/fdt088.

Browne J, Jamieson L, Lewsey J, van der Meulen J, Black N, Cairns J, Lamping D, Smith S, Copley L, Horrocks, J (2007) *Patient Reported Outcome Measures (PROMs) in Elective Surgery.* Report to the Department of Health. London: Health Services Research Unit, London School of Hygiene & Tropical Medicine and Clinical Effectiveness Unit, Royal College of Surgeons of England. Available at: www.lshtm.ac.uk/hsru/research/PROMs- Report-12-Dec-07.pdf (accessed 15 June, 2015).

Burström K, Johannesson M, Diderichsen F. (2001) Swedish population health-related quality of life results using the EQ-5D. *Quality of Life Research*, vol 10, no 7, pp 621–635.

Burström B, Burström K, Corman D (2014) *Livsvillkor, levnadsvanor och hälsa i Stockholms län – öppna jämförelser 2014.* (Living conditions, health-related behaviours and health in Stockholm County – open comparisons 2014.) Stockholm: Stockholms läns landsting, Centrum för epidemiologi och samhällsmedicin. Rapport 2014:3. (Stockholm: Stockholm County Council, 2014. Report 2014:3.) (In Swedish)

Chard J, Kuczawski M, Black N, van der Meulen J on behalf of the POiS (2011) Outcomes of elective surgery undertaken in independent sector treatment centres and NHS providers in England: audit of patient outcomes in surgery *British Medical Journal*, vol 343, d6404 doi: 10.1136/bmj.d6404

Coombes R (2008) Ahead of the game. *British Medical Journal*, vol 336, no 7659, p 1465.

Department of Health (2009) High Quality Care for All: Our journey so far. Department of Health, London. Available at: www.aemh.org/pdf/NextstageDarzireport.pdf (accessed 15 June, 2015).

Department of Health (2012) *Patient Reported Outcome Measures (PROMs) in England: The Case-Mix Adjustment Methodology.* London: Department of Health.

Foot C, Sonola L, Maybin J, Naylor C (2012) *Service-Line Management: Can it Improve Quality and Efficiency?* The King's Fund, London. Available at: www.kingsfund.org.uk/sites/files/kf/service-line-management-quality-efficiency-kings-fund-january2011.pdf (accessed 15 June, 2015).

Gutacker N, Bojke C, Daidone S, Devlin NJ, Parkin D, Street A (2013a) Truly inefficient or providing better quality of care?: Analysing the relationship between risk-adjusted hospital costs and patients' health outcomes. *Health Economics*, vol 22, no 8, pp 931–947. doi: 10.1002/hec.2871.

Gutacker N, Bojke C, Daidone S, Devlin N, Street A. (2013b) Hospital variation in patient reported outcomes at the level of EQ-5D dimensions: evidence from England. *Med Decis Making*, vol 33, no 6, pp 804–818. doi: 10.1177/0272989×13482523.

Health and Social Care Information Centre (2014) *Provisional Monthly Patient Reported Outcome Measures (PROMs) in England – April to March 2013, May 2014 release.* Leeds: HSCIC.

Jarman B, Gault S, Alves B, Hider A, Dolan S, Cook A, Hurwitz B, Iezzoni LI (1999) Explaining differences in English hospital death rates using routinely collected data. *BMJ*, vol 318: pp 1515–1520.

Neuburger J, Hutchings A, Allwood D, Black N, van der Meulen JH (2012) Sociodemographic differences in the severity and duration of disease amongst patients undergoing hip or knee replacement surgery. *J Public Health*, vol 34, pp 421–429.

NHS Choices (2015) *Quality Accounts.* Available at: www.nhs.uk/aboutNHSChoices/professionals/healthandcareprofessionals/quality-accounts/Pages/about-quality-accounts.aspx (accessed 15 June, 2015).

NHS England (2013) *Patient Reported Outcome Measures (PROMs): An alternative aggregation methodology for case-mix adjustment.* NHS England. Available at: www.england.nhs.uk/statistics/wp-content/uploads/sites/2/2013/07/proms-agg-meth-adju.pdf (accessed 15 June, 2015).

Nilsson E, Orwelius L, Kristenson M. (2015) Review: Patient reported outcomes (PRO) in the Swedish National Quality Registers. *JIM* (forthcoming)

Nuttall D, Parkin D, Devlin N (2013) Inter-provider comparison of patient reported outcomes: developing an adjustment to account for differences in patient case mix. *Health Economics*. doi: 10.1002/hec.2999

Rolfson O, Kärrholm J, Dahlberg LE, Garellick G. (2011) Patient reported outcomes in the Swedish Hip Arthroplasty Register: results of a nationwide prospective observational study. *J Bone Joint Surg Br*, vol 93, no 7, pp 867–875.

Sun S, Irestig R, Burström B, Beijer U, Burström K. (2012) Health-related quality of life (EQ-5D) among homeless persons compared to a general population sample in Stockholm County 2006. *Scandinavian Journal of Public Health*, vol 40, no 2, 115–125.

Vallance-Owen A (2008) Measuring patient care: PROMs promote health gain and patient involvement. *British Medical Journal*, vol 336, no 7640, p 344.

Vallance-Owen A, Cubbin S, Warren V, Matthews B (2004) Outcome monitoring to facilitate clinical governance; experience from a national programme in the independent sector. *Journal of Public Health* (Oxford), vol 26, no 2, pp 187–192.

Varagunam M, Hutchings A, Black N (2014) Do patient reported outcomes offer a more sensitive method for comparing the outcomes of consultants than mortality? A multilevel analysis of routine data *BMJ Qual Saf*, doi:10.1136/bmjqs-2014–003551/.

CHAPTER 6

Commissioners: quality, value for money and fairness

Health care systems around the world are organised in different ways, but all, to some degree or other, exercise commissioning or purchasing of health care on behalf of patients. Since the early 1990s, commissioners in the English NHS have purchased secondary care on behalf of their resident populations with the broad goals of ensuring a comprehensive set of services available to all in need while striving for best value for money from their allocated budgets. The current title given to commissioner organisations is the Clinical Commissioning Group (CCG), though the central NHS body, NHS England, commissions certain services directly.

PRO data can inform many of commissioners' key functions and activities, including:

- *monitoring the performance* of the providers they commission services from, specifying minimum performance on PROs via their contracts with those providers
- *incentivising providers* to improve patient health by linking payment to performance on PROs
- *prioritising spending* by using evidence on PROs *across* different service areas to inform decisions about how much the CCG should spend
- *benchmarking their own performance* against that of other commissioners, identifying which are most effective in commissioning improvements in patient health measured using PROs
- *monitoring (and acting on) inequitable variations* in patient health outcomes that are revealed when PRO data are examined by age, gender, sociodemographic characteristics and so on.

Broadly, commissioners must decide *what* to purchase, *who* to purchase it from and *how best* to purchase services. The potential for using PROs in economic evaluation concerns the first of these questions. But how might PROs be used to decide which providers to purchase services from; on what basis; and how to incentivise providers to lift their performance on PROs?

In this chapter, we begin by considering the opportunities and issues for commissioners using PRO data as a basis for assessing the value-for-money of the services they commission. We then discuss the role of PROs in commissioners' contracts with service providers to address ways of incentivising provider performance, and the benchmarking of performance with other commissioners.

Using Patient Reported Outcomes to Improve Health Care,
First Edition. John Appleby, Nancy Devlin and David Parkin.
© 2016 John Wiley & Sons, Ltd. Published 2016 by John Wiley & Sons, Ltd.

Value-for-money from commissioner budgets

Within any given budgetary period, the total NHS budget – and the budgets of each commissioner – available for spending on health care are fixed. The challenge for commissioners is to allocate that fixed budget among health care services so as to achieve, to the greatest possible extent, its goal of meeting the health care needs of its resident population.

The challenge for the budget-holder is to weigh up the costs and benefits of the services it could buy, and to allocate budgets among activities so as to maximise the overall improvement in health possible within the budget constraints. In practice, there is a wide range of complex national and local influences on commissioning, and cost-effectiveness may not be the principal (or even an important) consideration in how these choices are made at the local level (Williams *et al.*, 2008; Appleby *et al.*, 2009).

At present, the systematic use of economic evaluation is exemplified by the approach taken by NICE in its appraisal of (predominantly) new health care technologies. NICE's approach to weighing up benefits and costs relies on a particular form of cost-effectiveness analysis: benefits are measured as QALYs gained from treatment, and considered alongside the change in costs associated with that treatment. The focus is on the benefits and costs incremental to the existing treatment, and cost-effectiveness is captured by the incremental cost-effectiveness ratio (ICER), which shows the addition to cost per QALY gained.

The judgment about whether any given cost per QALY gained represents good value-for-money is made by comparison against a normative benchmark: the cost-effectiveness 'threshold'. This is in effect the price that NICE is willing to pay for one additional QALY. NICE intends this price to reflect the marginal cost of buying an additional QALY in the NHS, given its budget constraint. At present, NICE's guidelines are as follows:

- a treatment with a cost per QALY of less than £20 000 is considered to be clearly cost-effective
- if a treatment costs £20 000–30 000 per QALY, other sorts of benefits or considerations must be evident
- if a treatment costs more than £30 000 per QALY, an increasingly strong case needs to be made for the technology to be recommended (National Institute for Health and Clinical Excellence, 2013).

In practice, however, the NICE threshold seems to be much higher than these figures suggest. Dakin *et al.* (2014) have estimated that on average it is only when a treatment exceeds £40 000 per QALY gained that it is more likely that NICE will reject rather than accept it.

NICE's approach is far from perfect: QALYs capture only part of the benefits that result from health and health care; and the threshold that is crucial to its decisions lacks a basis in evidence. However, it is the best example both within the NHS, and arguably internationally, of an attempt to make difficult resource allocation decisions in health care in a way that is explicit, transparent and based on sound economic principles.

Partly because of this and partly because denying access to a new health care technology is often controversial, NICE's decisions can be contentious. But the products and technologies available to NHS patients in England and Wales as a result of NICE's decisions over more than a decade so far account for less than 10% of total NHS spending, which raises an interesting question: what is known about the value-for-money of the *other* 90%?

While some evidence exists, the majority seems to focus on new treatments or technologies. In part, this is because new technologies tend to be expensive, and so are an obvious focus for decision makers; and it is also because the availability of data from clinical trials more readily facilitates sophisticated and interesting (to economists!) analyses than does the sort of administrative and observational data available on existing services. The result is that the effectiveness and cost-effectiveness of much of what is done routinely in the NHS remains unknown. Some services, for some patients, may be very poor value-for-money. Finding out more about these and reallocating money toward services that *are* cost-effective could yield substantial improvements in patient health from existing budgets.

PROs and commissioning

These are, of course, matters of considerable interest to the people who hold the budgets in the NHS and other health systems: the commissioners. The decisions made every day by commissioners in purchasing health care for their communities result in a particular allocation of resources and a corresponding aggregate improvement in, and distribution of, health. But, unless health is measured in some way, commissioners will not know what outcomes result from a given set of commissioned services – and whether commissioning a different set of services would be better overall.

PROs have a potentially very important role to play in helping commissioners make sure they are getting good value-for-money. The current Department of Health PROMs programme in the NHS in England includes, as noted earlier, both condition-specific and generic measures. The generic instrument being used – the EQ-5D – has two features that make it particularly useful in the context of commissioning.

First, because it describes health in a general way, it facilitates comparisons of health improvements across dissimilar illnesses and treatments. This is critical to assessments of value-for-money, because weighing up benefits and costs necessarily involves assessing health improvements in one area of health care versus deterioration in health elsewhere.

Second, as discussed in Chapters 2 and 7, use of the EQ-5D to calculate QALYs for use in cost-effectiveness studies means that the methods are broadly comparable with those used in evidence submitted to NICE.

At present the PRO data are available only to the NHS in England for a small set of elective surgical procedures. But if the collection of PRO data is rolled out across more conditions and are embedded in most health service delivery, it will be possible to analyse these data at a number of levels. For example:

- PRO data could be examined alongside programme budgeting data to look for high-level *disparities in the value yielded from commissioner allocations* of resources between programme budgets
- it would be possible to examine *how levels of spending relate to health outcomes* for patients in each programme budget area
- the analysis can also drill down to look at the *value-for-money of particular services and particular providers*
- alternatively, drilling down still further, it would be possible to investigate *differences in the effects of treatment* on different patient sub-groups, and the comparative effectiveness of different ways of delivering services.

Using PROs to choose providers and manage performance

The presentation of comparative information of provider performance on PROs – such as the benchmarking shown in, for example, Figures 2.5, 3.3 and 3.4 in Chapters 2 and 3, – clearly has the scope to be used by commissioners in monitoring performance, setting minimum performance standards and selecting high-performing providers.

Just as there is a need to establish what sort of comparative information on provider performance is relevant to patients, similarly there is a need to know which form of analyses and reporting are most useful to commissioners in discharging their commissioning role. For example, while variation around the average performance may be of most relevance to patients, the identification of performance that falls below some acceptable minimum standard might be of greater interest to commissioners. Quite what such standards should be – where, literally, to draw the lower bounds on funnel plots for instance – is difficult to say. However, as with the treatment and provider choices facing individual patients, there is a degree of uncertainty surrounding patient reported outcome measures.

One way in which commissioners will be affected by PROs is via patients voting with their feet and choosing providers that perform well on PRO-based indicators. Under payment systems (such as Payment by Results) where money follows the patient – the corresponding revenue flows from commissioners to providers creates indirect incentives for providers to improve their performance on PROs. However, commissioners can also employ more direct means of linking payment to performance. For example, the English NHS has experimented with tying a proportion of a contract value to measures of health care quality – for example, the Commissioning for Quality and Innovation (CQUIN) payments scheme (Department of Health, 2008).

As data and knowledge around normal or expected variance in provider performance on PROs grows, commissioners will be able to sharpen up the use of incentive schemes to reward directly good performance from providers. In the absence of those data, commissioners are cautiously using PROs as part of their CQUIN payments.

Equitable health outcomes?

As we noted earlier, a key concern for commissioners of health care is not just the utilitarian objective of maximising value for money from their spending, but also with variations in access to, and use of, health services. This is especially the case in health systems such as the English NHS, organised on the basis of universal access, regardless of ability to pay. But to what extent has such access translated into equality of health outcomes? The collection of PRO data has allowed researchers to examine the correlations between systematic variations in health outcomes across socioeconomic dimensions such as income, class and more general measures of deprivation.

As Figure 6.1 shows, there seems to be a relationship between the pre-operative health state of patients and the level of socioeconomic deprivation in the areas in which they live. Patients from more deprived areas tend to have a lower level of health-related quality of life just prior to their operation for hernias or hip replacement than those living in less deprived areas.

Jenny Neuberger and colleagues have also found that even after adjusting pre-operative disease-specific measures for hip replacements (using the Oxford Hip Score) for a range of possibly confounding factors such as other existing medical problems, the difference in pre-operative health status, although small, persisted – with patients living in the most deprived areas being admitted to hospital for a hip replacement being in significantly worse health than those from the least deprived areas (Neuburger et al., 2012). Further, Neuburger et al. concluded that the symptoms of patients from more deprived areas tended to be more severe and more longstanding and that this was also the case for South Asian and black groups compared to white patients.

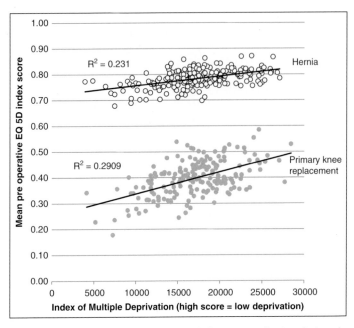

Figure 6.1 Socioeconomic deprivation and health state before operation (hernia and primary knee replacement): English hospitals: April–November 2010. Source: Authors' calculations

References

Appleby J, Devlin N, Parkin D, Buxton M, Chalkidou K (2009) Searching for cost effectiveness thresholds in the NHS. *Health Policy*, vol 91, no 3, pp 239–245.

Dakin H, Devlin N, Feng Y, Rice N, O'Neill P, Parkin D (2014) The influence of cost-effectiveness and other factors on NICE decisions. *Health Economics*. 10.1002/hec.3086.

Department of Health (2008) *Using the Commissioning for Quality and Innovation (CQUIN) Payment Framework*. For the NHS in England 2009/10. Available at: http://webarchive. nationalarchives.gov.uk/20130107105354/www.dh.gov.uk/en/Publicationsandstatistics/ Publications/PublicationsPolicyAndGuidance/DH_091443 (accessed on 1 July 2015).

National Institute for Health and Care Excellence (2013) *Guide to the Methods of Technology Appraisal 2013*. Available at: http://publications.nice.org.uk/pmg9 (accessed 15 June, 2015).

Neuburger J, Hutchings A, Allwood D, Black N, van der Meulen JH (2012) Sociodemographic differences in the severity and duration of disease amongst patients undergoing hip or knee replacement surgery. *J Public Health*, vol 34, pp 421–429.

Williams I, McIver S, Moore D, Bryan S (2008) The use of economic evaluations in NHS decision-making: a review and empirical investigation. *Health Technology Assessment*, vol 12, no 7, pp 1–175.

CHAPTER 7

Regulation, value for money and productivity

Two important issues that concern the users and payers of any health care service are quality assurance and value for money of the health care provided. These concerns extend beyond insuring that specific health care interventions and, more broadly, that services are safe to include the quality, cost effectiveness and productivity of health services. How might patient reported outcomes help with such issues? In particular, how can they play a part in the systematic regulation of health care, evaluation of its cost effectiveness and productivity?

Patient reported outcomes and regulation of health care

Given the nature of health care and, in particular, the potentially fatal consequences that could arise from the information asymmetry between providers and consumers, significant regulation of the health care industry is common in most countries. The scope of regulation – from requirements to register with a central authority in order to practice or trade, to regular inspections and requirements to meet minimum standards – varies between countries and over time.

For example, in England over the past decade, the scale and methods of regulating health care organisations to ensure safety and quality has undergone enormous change. The Care Quality Commission (CQC) now succeeds and subsumes previous organisations, namely the Healthcare Commission, the Commission for Social Care Inspection and the Mental Health Act Commission. The key aim of the CQC is 'to make sure better care is provided for everyone, whether that's in hospital, in care homes, in people's own homes, or elsewhere' (Care Quality Commission, 2009b).

Apart from changes in the regulatory structures, the way health care organisations are regulated and the data employed to do this have also changed. The CQC's initial measures to assess the quality of care provided by acute trusts applied to 2008–2009 and covered seven domains, such as safety and patient focus. Within each domain, more detailed measures and indicators were also assessed. The eventual composite assessment of a Trust's level of quality (excellent, good, fair or weak) also included its performance on 23 'national priorities' and 'existing commitments', such as cancer treatment waiting times, stroke care, incidence of *Clostridium difficile*, experience of patients and total time spent in accident and emergency departments. Within these aspects of performance are further aspects or indicators for each particular priority or commitment.

Using Patient Reported Outcomes to Improve Health Care,
First Edition. John Appleby, Nancy Devlin and David Parkin.
© 2016 John Wiley & Sons, Ltd. Published 2016 by John Wiley & Sons, Ltd.

Of note was the focus on measures of *process* rather than *outcome* in this assessment of quality of care, and furthermore, the reliance on indirect measures of quality. In terms of patients' own views and assessments, while elements of the national patient survey data were included, there was little direct input from patients on the quality of the care they received and no information on their health-related quality of life.

However, under the terms of the Health and Social Care Act 2008, from April 2010 this system of regulation and assessment changed to include a registration requirement for all health care providers coupled with inspections and special investigations by the CQC.

In its guidance on compliance with the act (Care Quality Commission, 2009a), the CQC noted that its approach to registration would draw on the experience of people using services by, among other things, '…defining quality in terms of *outcomes* wherever possible' (p. 6), and '…frequently and regularly using *information on the views and experiences of those using services* and their families and carers' (p. 6) (our emphasis). Furthermore, the CQC will check that providers '…obtain the views from the people who use their services to understand the quality of people's experiences' (p. 12). Finally, in terms of monitoring and reporting of the quality of services used by patients, health care organisations will be required to (among other things):

- Have appropriate systems for gathering, recording and evaluating accurate information about the quality and safety of the service, in particular people's experiences of the care, treatment and support they receive and its outcomes.
- Gather information about the safety and quality of their service from all relevant sources, including feedback from people using services, audits, adverse events, complaints, claims and other comments received.
- Use the findings from clinical audits, including those undertaken at a national level, and national service reviews to ensure that action is taken to protect people from risks associated with unsafe care, treatment and support.
- Use the information gathered to set goals about how the service can improve the quality and safety of experience for people who use services in order to comply with the Health and Social Care Act 2008 (Registration Requirements) Regulations 2009. (Care Quality Commission, 2009, pp. 77–78)

The emphasis on patients' own views, assessments and experience, and the focus on providers collecting and reporting on quality (i.e. outcomes) in this revised registration and inspection regime suggest that patient-reported outcome measures have an important potential role for the CQC. And indeed, more recent changes to the way the CQC assess the quality of health care organisations services includes an aggregating evaluation based on a wide range of clinical, staffing, and other indicators – including performance based on the routine PRO data collected for hip and knee replacement, groin hernia repairs and varicose vein procedures. An example of the indicators collated and assessed for one hospital – The Royal Bournemouth and Christchurch Hospitals NHS Foundation Trust – as part of the CQC's 'Intelligent Monitoring' reports in July 2014 shows, for example, that this hospital had an amber risk rating on PROs for knee replacements (Care Quality Commission, 2014).

The evaluation and monitoring of hospital performance is an international issue. As Jiaying Chen and Yaling Yang note (Box 7.1) China has begun a 4-year project (starting in 2015) to develop a framework to incorporate PROs, patient experience and satisfaction data for use in evaluating the performance of Chinese public hospitals.

Box 7.1 Application of PROs in China: progress, challenges and outlook

Jiaying Chen[1], Yaling Yang[2]

Although PROs have been used to evaluate health interventions in China for more than 15 years, these data were generally limited to research activities. There were some clinical trials using health related quality of life (HRQoL) questionnaires to evaluate treatments or therapies. Some pharmaceutical manufacturers also adopted HRQoL as the indicator of effects of new medicines. In 2008, the EQ-5D measure was introduced to the National Household Health Survey (NHSS) to measure the health related quality of life of the Chinese population and has been included by NHSS since then. Value sets of the Chinese version of EQ-5D–3L were developed recently.

Researchers and health officials have started to explore the indicators of PROs to evaluate health programmes, such as chronic disease management and elderly people's health management. Recently, the EQ-5D–3L was included in a large scale health program aiming to improve primary health care access in rural china (Ningxia Project, 2015). Overall, however, the use of PROs to assess health care system and aid decision making has been somewhat limited in China.

China's ongoing reform on health care system highlights the changes in managing systems and operating mechanisms. Evaluation of performance of health care providers usually focuses on optimising service procedures and standardising medical practices. As a result, instead of outputs and outcomes, process and activities are currently the major areas for appraisal in order to improve quality and efficiency of health care.

Currently, PROs, patients' satisfaction and experiences are often mixed by Chinese researchers and health managerial officials. Observed changes in self-reported health before and after a treatment could be used to assess provider performance, but experiences alone might not be adequate to indicate hospital performance – potentially confounding with different expectations between people. Both researchers and officials in China have emphasised the use of indicators of patients' satisfaction with service received as part of hospital performance. However, those indicators do not cover all aspects of patient's experiences or outcomes. And local health authorities have not yet established strict monitoring mechanism to guarantee the accountability of data collected.

'People-centred services' has long been a stated national policy, and patients and their needs and demands are now the universal target for health authorities and health institutions at all levels to meet. Backed by strong political will and firm national determination, more and more researchers and health officials are aware of the importance of PROs in health service evaluation. Further, with IT infrastructure well-developed in many areas, the implementation of PROs collection and processing should advance and become more systematic in the future.

Recently, a 4-year project (starting in 2015) has been funded by the Chinese National Science Fund to develop a framework to incorporate PROs, patient's experience and satisfaction data for use in evaluating the performance of Chinese public hospitals adopting different reform strategies. This is an important initiate to evaluate hospital performance from the patient's perspective. There are challenges however. PROs and other patient-derived measures need to be defined and assessed in China's context. Decisions need to be made about which outcome measures to use in for example primary health facilities and hospitals. There is some way to go in setting up the systems to collect and analyse such data. In addition, both generic and disease-specific instruments need to be selected or adapted, piloted and rolled out in line with China's culture and context. Finally, incentive mechanisms (e.g. pay for performance, results-based financing etc.) linking PROs results to improved hospital performance need to be designed. External evaluation of this work will be commissioned and published during the course of the project.

[1] *Nanjing Medical University.* [2] *University of Oxford.*

Using PRO data to measure cost-effectiveness

Because they incorporate quality of life information, PROs can be used to estimate changes in Quality Adjusted Life Years, permitting calculation of the cost-effectiveness ratio favoured by NICE for its decision making, the cost per QALY gained. Using this approach, Appleby *et al.* (2013) were able to confirm the findings based on clinical trials that hip replacements are in general good value for money, at an average of £1200–2100 per QALY gained, compared with the official NICE criterion of £20 000 – see Chapter 5. (Further details of how these figures were calculated are given later.) However, they also found that the cost per QALY gained varied considerably over providers, with the highest 9–10 times greater than the lowest. This was attributable almost entirely to variations in cost, showing again little or no relationship between costs and outcomes. Pennington *et al.* (2013) used the same PRO hip replacement data to compare the relative cost-effectiveness of different prostheses, finding that for most patient groups hybrid are the most cost effective and cementless the least. A similar analysis has also been carried out for hernia repairs by Coronini-Cronberg *et al.* (2013), who were also able to compare the cost-effectiveness of laparoscopic and open surgery.

The inclusion of the EQ-5D in the NHS PROMs programme is useful for a number of reasons, including the fact that it is designed to facilitate economic evaluations. It is accompanied by a social value set (Dolan, 1997) that makes straightforward the estimation of QALY gains. The EQ-5D is already widely used in cost-effectiveness analysis in the United Kingdom – indeed, it is the instrument recommended for use in evidence submitted to NICE (NICE, 2013). A simple explanation of how EQ-5D health states are valued and used in the estimation of QALYs is given in Box 7.2.

Box 7.2 Valuing EQ-5D PROMs data

For the purposes of economic evaluation, standard methods of analysis typically rely on data from the first part of the EQ-5D, where patients tick boxes to describe their health in terms of five dimensions (mobility, self-care, usual activities, pain/discomfort and anxiety/depression) and three (or, five, using the latest EQ-5D–5L questionnaire) levels.

For the three-level EQ-5D, no problem on a dimension is coded as '1', some problems as '2' and extreme problems as '3'. As an example, consider a patient who has no mobility problems, some self-care problems, extreme problems with usual activities and severe pain or discomfort, but is not anxious or depressed. Recording these in the order the dimensions appear, this health state is '12331' – this is simply a shorthand way of describing this particular state. The three-level EQ-5D describes 243 ($=3^5$) possible health states, from 11111 (full health) to 33333 (extreme problems on each dimension).

To use these data in the estimation of QALYs, the health states need to be summarised by a single index number. To do this requires a quality of life 'weight' for each state. These weights (also referred to as utilities or values) are meant to reflect the opinions of the general public about what it would be like living with these health problems. A UK social value set is available for all 243 states, obtained from responses to questions asked of a large, representative sample of the general public (Dolan, 1997; Szende et al., 2007). These are the values used by NICE in assessing cost-effectiveness.

These values are on a scale from 1 (the value assigned to full health) through to 0 (dead), with values less than zero reflecting health states considered worse than being dead.

For example, the UK value for health state 12331 is 0.07 – this means that 10 years lived in that state is considered 'worth' just 0.7 of a year of full health (i.e. 0.7 of a QALY). In this case, the low value is particularly influenced by there being extreme problems on two dimensions, with one of these being pain/discomfort. A value of 1.0 means that 10 years living in that state is equal to 10 years full health, whereas a value of 0 would imply that 10 years lived in that state would equal zero QALYs.

Value sets for the 3125 ($=5^5$) states described by the EQ-5D-5L (see Appendix 2) are currently being developed for a range of countries, including England (see Devlin et al. 2015), Canada, Spain, The Netherlands, Japan, South Korea, Thailand and many more.

Box 7.3 shows how PRO data can be used to calculate a cost per QALY. While arithmetically straightforward, there are limitations to such calculations, which are discussed in the following.

Box 7.3 Calculating cost per QALY gained using PROMs data: hip replacement

Part 1: the benefits

Orthopaedic surgery does not generally improve patients' length of life except in very rare cases, so the gain in patients' QALYs arises from improvements in the *quality* of their remaining life years. Health-related quality of life is likely to be affected by joint problems in a number of ways. The most obvious would be limitations on mobility and the ability to engage in usual activities, plus the experience of pain or discomfort. Other, less obvious, aspects of health might also be affected by joint problems, and improved by surgery. For example, Devlin et al. (2010) showed that problems with anxiety/depression are very commonly reported by those awaiting hip replacement and that alleviating this is also an important source of improvement in quality of life following surgery.

Appleby et al. (2013) used English hospital-level EQ-5D data before and after hip replacement surgery for 2009–2010 covering over 26 000 patients, together with assumptions about the time over which to calculate the average number of QALYs generated and about the change in QALYs if no operation was performed (the counterfactual) to estimate, for each hospital, the benefits of hip replacement as measured by the average change in QALYs relative to no treatment.

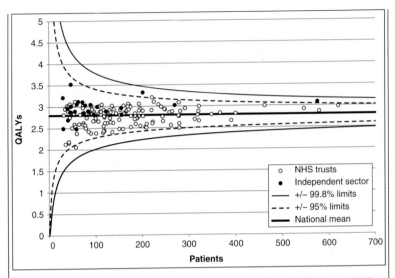

Figure 7.1 QALY change following a hip operation: English hospitals (April 2009–August 2010) Source: Appleby *et al.* (2013) Reproduced with permission of Sage Publications.

The average 'life' of an artificial joint was taken to be 15 years, and this was used the relevant period of time for the estimation of the benefit of surgery. The overall QALY change is the difference between the before and after value for each hospital over and above the change in QALYs assumed if no operation was performed on patients. Figure 7.1 shows the spread of these changes in the form of a funnel plot. On average there was an increase of around 2.7 QALYs per patient, ranging from around 2 to 3.5.

In broad terms, hip operations seem to provide fairly good benefits to patients. And while there is some variation between hospitals, these are mostly within acceptable limits. However, a crucial question for commissioners is the cost of obtaining such benefits: are hip operations good value for money?

Part 2: the costs and effects

Data on the costs of individual hospital procedures has been calculated and collated for English hospitals since the late 1990s. Using this National Reference Costs data for those types of hip operations included as part of the national PROMs scheme together with the QALY estimates detailed here, it is straightforward to compute a cost per QALY for each hospital.

Figure 7.2 shows the results in the form of a cost-effectiveness 'plane' for NHS hospitals only (there are no public data on costs for independent sector hospitals treating patients paid for by the NHS). Each point on the plane is one hospital, and the scattering of these points indicates the variation between hospitals in terms of the changes in health (shown on the horizontal axis). The vertical axis shows the cost of the treatment, which across all NHS hospitals in 2009–2010 was £5800 – but varied considerably.

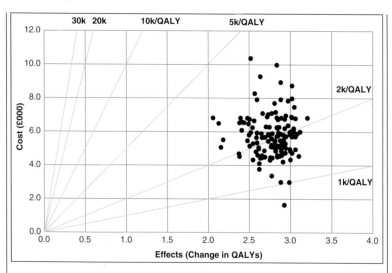

Figure 7.2 Cost-effectiveness plane for hip replacement surgery: English hospitals (April 2009–August 2010). Source: Appleby *et al.* (2013) Reproduced with permission of Sage Publications.

The rays from the origin represent various levels of cost per QALY – from £1000 to £30 000. On average, the cost per QALY across all English hospitals was around £2100.

Taken at face value, the results suggest that – notwithstanding the variation between individual patients' baseline and post-surgery PROMs – overall, orthopaedic surgery is extremely good value-for-money. The average gain in QALYs for these patients was 5.2, that is, each patient gained an average of 5.2 years in full health as a result of the surgery. The cost-effectiveness ratio – the average cost and average gain in QALYs – is just £1800 – much lower than the threshold range of £20 000–30 000 per QALY that NICE claims that it uses as its criterion in assessing value-for-money.

There are, however, some important limitations to using EQ-5D data from the PROMs programme in these ways. In particular, there are challenges in applying the standard methods of economic evaluation to PRO data because they are *observational* in nature. The key problem in using simple after-minus-before PRO data to estimate gains in QALYs is that it takes no account of the counterfactual: that is, what would have happened to the patient if he or she had not had the surgery?

The major limitations to these cost-effectiveness estimates are:

- It is not possible to be certain that the quality of life reported after surgery is *caused* by that surgery. Other things might have happened – to patients' general health, other conditions they suffer from, or their life circumstances – that could either improve or worsen self-reported health as captured by PROs. These need to be controlled for.
- Inferring the benefit of treatment from just two observations of PROs makes the timing of the second observation crucial. For example, collecting PRO data 6 months after hip surgery might miss the time when patients first get back to their usual activities, as well as giving no real indication of the longer-term outcomes and their durability.

- In the examples described in Box 7.2, only the cost of the surgery itself was taken into account. Without surgery, patients might have required increasing levels of pain and symptom relief, mobility aids and supportive care services. After surgery, patients might also require help with pain control, physiotherapy assistance with regaining full mobility and so on. The relevant costs are the *net incremental* costs, in relation to the relevant comparator. Again, the issue with PRO data is that we do not know what the comparator is for these patients. In effect, all of these issues link to the nature of the data:
- There is a limited number of observations at one point in time from which to extrapolate quality of life changes over time
- There is uncertainty about the relevant counterfactual
- Other, unobserved, factors that are not controlled for also exert an influence.

These problems are important, but are they insurmountable? The issues involved in using observational data in economic evaluation are well known (Drummond, 1998) and there are means of addressing them. For example, clinical evidence and clinical consensus panels can be used to construct appropriate counterfactuals. Factors that might bias results, such as co-morbidities or patients' general health, can be controlled for. Although PRO data cannot reveal the future prospects for patients receiving treatment now, the same limitation applies to data obtained in the context of clinical trials of new medicines and modelling techniques offer a means of addressing this source of uncertainty. And PRO data do have the important advantage of reflecting actual patient experience of real health service delivery – in comparison with clinical trials, which are often undertaken under conditions that are not typical of normal practice.

Notwithstanding the limitations of PRO data, they represent a hugely valuable source of evidence that will help to establish – in many cases, for the first time – whether health care services are effective and good value for money. Even rudimentary analyses may be broadly informative and identify areas of service delivery and spending where there are large disparities in cost-effectiveness across programmes. The relevant question is not 'How does an economic evaluation based on PRO data compare with a perfect economic evaluation study?', but rather, 'Is an economic evaluation based on PRO data, even if imperfect, better than having no evidence at all?'

Although there are problems with using PRO data to undertake economic evaluation, there are still some ways in which these data can be used immediately to strengthen some technical aspects of health technology appraisal, such as the following:

- They can provide a source of typical patient outcomes and values for different diseases/conditions so as to allow better economic modelling of new interventions. The size of the data sets that will be generated in the NHS means it will be possible to examine the impact on disutility of diseases by patient characteristics (such as age) or when experienced alongside specific combinations and severities of co-morbidities and so on. It is not generally possible to obtain these insights within the context of clinical trials, in which the numbers are relatively small.
- They can permit detailed analysis of the relationship between the EQ-5D and the disease-specific measures.
- They begin to identify interventions or sub-groups of patients in which/for whom apparent benefits of interventions are less than had been expected, and that might be justified by costs. PRO data can serve to identify topics where further investigation is required; and which can then be the subject of a more formal assessment (where data are obtained both on the treatment and the counterfactual).

Key to the wider use of PROs in assessing value for money will be the development of economic evaluation and statistical methods that take into account the observational nature of the data noted previously, in a manner that is robust and facilitates legitimate comparisons of value-for-money across dissimilar conditions and treatments.

Measuring NHS output and productivity

While data on PROs are starting to find their way into the battery of indicators of quality used to assess hospitals in England and have the potential to assess cost effectiveness from real-world data, there is another aspect of performance across the whole system which has over recent years grappled with the problem of what measures to use to reflect the quality of health care services, namely, productivity.

Measuring the output of the health care services (indeed, any industry, public or private) is a difficult task. Although conceptually straightforward – productivity is the amount of output for a given level of input – in practice, calculating such an apparently simple ratio is rather hard. Traditionally, the UK Office for National Statistics has measured the output part of the productivity ratio for the NHS in the form of a cost-weighted activity index, where cost is used as a substitute for price and all the various activities of the NHS – inpatients, outpatients, prescriptions and so on – are added together using their shares of the total spend on the NHS as weights. The implication is that costs reflect the values society places on the activities carried out by the NHS. Dividing changes in this index from year to year by changes in total spending provides a measure of the change in productivity. On this basis, the most recent estimates of NHS productivity by the Office for National Statistics (ONS) suggest that between 1995 and 2012, the productivity of the NHS across the UK rose by an average of 0.8% per year (ONS, 2015).

Although there have been developments in the number and type of activities included in the cost-weighted activity index to make the measure more sensitive to changes over time in the mix of activities carried out by the NHS, and while the productivity estimate quoted earlier includes some adjustment for the quality of the health 'product', there remains scope for improving the way quality is accounted for.

Historically, no account was taken of changes in the quality of the outputs produced by the NHS[4]. The implicit assumption was that the NHS made no progress over time in the quality of, say, hip replacements and that the quality of such procedures is the same regardless of the surgeon or hospital. It is as if the output of the computer industry is calculated simply by counting the number of machines produced, ignoring the improvements in memory and processing power of computers over time.

A key recommendation of the Atkinson Review (Atkinson, 2005) was that the output of the NHS (and indeed that of all public services) should be adjusted for quality. Failure to do so could mean that where quality improves and leads, for example, to a reduction in the amount of activity necessary to achieve a given outcome, it would appear that output, as measured by the cost-weighted activity index, had reduced and also that productivity (also based on the relatively crude cost-weighted activity measure) would also appear to have fallen, providing a misleading picture of the actual change. Specifically, Atkinson suggested that NHS activities could be marked up or down by a percentage point reflecting indicators of success and the contribution of the service to that success.

---

[4] Indeed, for many years there was an assumption that the output of the NHS always equalled its input; even if the NHS improved its productivity this would not be revealed in the ratio of outputs to inputs by definition!

Various attempts have been made to adjust NHS output for changes in the quality of the product. For example, researchers at York University and the National Institute of Economic and Social Research (NIESR) constructed an alternative to the cost-weighted activity index using weights based on waiting times and change in health status of patients. Taking three illustrative procedures and using actual cost, waiting time and health outcome data, they found that weighting coronary bypass surgery activity in terms of the change in QALYs that such procedures generated led to smaller increases in the activity index than the weighting for cost. However, the reverse was the case for hip replacements and upper genital tract procedures (Dawson *et al.*, 2005). The basis for the 'Q' in QALY used in the York example was an EQ-5D index score.

The ONS has also attempted to adjust NHS outputs for quality using a range of measures suggested by the York/NIESR team (Carless, 2008). Overall, adjustments for quality factors such as reduced waiting times, changes in heart attack survival and improvements in patient experience, increased the level of NHS output and productivity by around 0.5 percentage points per year over the period 2003–2004 to 2010–2011 (see Figure 7.3).

There has been broad agreement among those investigating ways to improve the measurement of the outputs and productivity of the NHS that changes in patients' health status would be a desirable quality adjustment. So far, the problem has been the lack of any data directly bearing on this. However, the EQ-5D data now being generated through patient-reported outcome measures can be used not only to monitor quality-adjusted output and productivity at the level of individual procedures and health care organisations, but also changes in these measures over time. An example of the difference adjusting for quality using EQ-5D data can make is illustrated in Box 7.4.

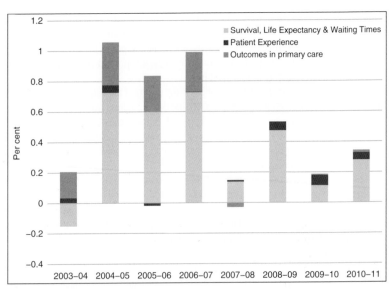

Figure 7.3 Contribution to NHS output growth of the quality adjustment factor 2003–2004 to 2010–2011. Source: Data: ONS (2012)

Box 7.4 A better way of measuring NHS output?

Pritchard (2004) provides an example of the way that relative costs are used in the construction of output measures, using knee replacement and varicose vein procedures.

Categories of treatments and activities	Year 1 unit cost £	Year 1 expenditure £m	Year 1 expenditure shares	Year 1 activities	Year 2 activities	Index 1999–2000	Index 2000–2001	Percentage growth 2000–2001
Illustration of detailed calculation (method used from June 2004)								
Knee replacement	4,785	165.9	0.833	34 662	39 902	100	115.1	15.1
Varicose vein procedure	835	33.3	0.167	39 923	42 150	100	105.6	5.6
Total		1992.2	1.000	74 585	82 052	100	113.5	13.5
Illustration of *unweighted* calculation (method used from June 2004)								
Total				74 585	82 052	100	110	10.0

Source: Pritchard (2004). Office for National Statistics licensed under the Open Government Licence v.3.0.

The table shows that weighting by cost produces a measured increase in output of 13.5%, whereas no weighting suggests an increase of 10.0%.

However, the cost-weighted calculation relies on the strong assumption that the cost of each procedure is a reflection of the value these interventions provide to patients, with knee replacements being valued at five times more than varicose vein procedures.

PROMs provide an alternative means of assessing the relative value of these interventions. For example, we could base the 'weight' to be applied to the two sorts of operations on the relative value of the health improvement resulting from them.

	Mean pre-operative EQ-5D index	Mean post-operative EQ-5D index	Change in utility
Knee replacement	0.39	0.70	0.31
Varicose vein procedures	0.76	0.87	0.11

Source: extracted from Browne *et al.* (2007).
Note: the figures show the average values (utilities) for the EQ-5D profiles reported by patients in the PROMs pilot study before and after surgery.

This would suggest that, on average, the value of the improvement in health resulting from a knee replacement is 2.82 times greater than that from a varicose veins procedure. Factoring this into the activity, these figures suggest a percentage increase in output of around 12.5%. This is lower than the cost-weighted estimate, but higher than the unweighted estimate. Knee replacements cost more than varicose veins *and* produce much greater increases in health-related quality of life, but using the relative share of total expenditure as the basis for the weight applied to each exaggerates the relative value of the health improvement from knee replacement.

Clearly, for the English NHS, the current scope of the PRO data set only covers a small fraction of its total activities and will have a marginal impact on the overall measure of outputs and productivity. Nevertheless, there is the prospect of using this data in combination with the traditional cost-weighted activity measure and expanding the use of PROs as a quality adjustment.

A remaining challenge, noted by the Office of Health Economics Commission on NHS Outcomes, Performance and Productivity (Office of Health Economics, 2008), is the importance of being able to link health outcomes to the delivery of complete treatments, packages or pathways of care, rather than its individual components.

Ultimately, the availability of routinely collected PRO data, as well as programme budget data for each primary care trust creates an important opportunity to link costs, activity and outcomes that '…will offer the NHS a powerful tool to assess overall performance and to understand key areas for change' (Office of Health Economics, 2008, p. 59).

References

Appleby J, Poteliakhoff E, Shah K, Devlin N. (2013) Using patient-reported outcome measures to estimate cost-effectiveness of hip replacements in English hospitals. *J R Soc Med*, vol 106, no 8, pp 323–331.

Atkinson A (2005) *Atkinson Review: Final Report. Measurement of Government Output and Productivity for the National Accounts*. Basingstoke: Palgrave MacMillan.

Care Quality Commission (2009a) *Guidance about Compliance with the Health and Social Care Act 2008 (Registration Requirements) Regulations 2009: Draft guidance*. London: Care Quality Commission. Available at: http://apps.bps.org.uk/_publicationfiles/consultation-responses/CQC%20Registration%20-%20draft%20guidance.pdf (accessed on 1 July 2015).

Care Quality Commission (2009b) *Who We Are*. Care Quality Commission website. Available at: www.cqc.org.uk/content/who-we-are (accessed 15 June, 2015).

Care Quality Commission (2014) *Intelligent Monitoring Report on the Royal Bournemouth and Christchurch Hospitals NHS Foundation Trust, July 2014*. CQC, London. Available at: www.cqc.org.uk/sites/default/files/RDZ_103v3_WV.pdf (accessed 15 June, 2015).

Carless E (2008) *Adjusting Measures of Public Service Output for Quality of Service*. Newport: UK Centre for the Measurement of Government Activity, Office for National Statistics. Available at: Carless E (2008) Adjusting Measures of Public Service Output for Quality of Service. Newport: UK Centre for the Measurement of Government Activity, Office for National Statistics www.ons.gov.uk/ons/guide-method/ukcemga/publications (accessed 1 July 2015).

Coronini-Cronberg S, Appleby J, Thompson J. (2013) Application of patient-reported outcome measures (PROMs) data to estimate cost-effectiveness of hernia surgery in England. *J R Soc Med*, vol 106, no 7, pp 278–287.

Dawson D, Gravelle H, O'Mahony M, Street A, Weale M, Castelli A, Jacobs R, Kind P, Loveridge P, Martin S, Stevens P, Stokes L (2005) *Developing New Approaches to Measuring NHS Outputs and Activity*. Centre for Health Economics Research Paper 6. York: University of York. Available at: www.york.ac.uk/inst/che/pdf/rp6.pdf (accessed 15 June, 2015).

Devlin N, Parkin D, Browne J (2010) Patient Reported Outcome Measures in the NHS: new methods for analysing and reporting EQ-5D data. *Health Economics*, vol 19, pp 886–905.

Devlin, N, Shah, K., Feng, Y, Mulhern, B., van Hout B (2015) An EQ-5D-5L value set for England. *OHE Research Papers*, Vol. 15, no 3 (forthcoming) www.ohe.org/publications.

Dolan P (1997) Modelling valuations for EuroQol health states. *Medical Care*, vol 35, no 11, pp 1095–1108.

Drummond MF (1998) Experimental versus observational data in the economic evaluation of pharmaceuticals. *Medical Decision Making*, vol 18, no 2 (suppl), pp S12–S18.

National Institute for Health and Care Excellence (2013) *Guide to the Methods of Technology Appraisal 2013*. Available at: http://publications.nice.org.uk/pmg9 (accessed 15 June, 2015).

Ningxia Project, (2015) Re-alignment of Health System Incentives to Improve Affordable and Effective Healthcare Project. Available at http://www.bsg.ox.ac.uk/research/projects/re-alignment-health-system-incentives.

Office of Health Economics (2008) *Report of the Office of Health Economics Commission on NHS Outcomes, Performance and Productivity*. London: Office of Health Economics.

Office for National Statistics (ONS) (2012) *Public Service Productivity Estimates: Health care*: 2010 Office for National Statistics, Cardiff. Available at: www.ons.gov.uk/ons/dcp171766_289768.pdf (accessed 15 June, 2015).

Office for National Statistics (ONS) (2015) *Public Service Productivity Estimates: Health care*. Office for National Statistics, Cardiff. Available at: www.ons.gov.uk/ons/rel/psa/public-sector-productivity-estimates–healthcare/2012/art-healthcare.html (accessed 1 July, 2015).

Pennington M, Grieve R, Sekhon JS, Gregg P, Black N, van der Meulen JH. (2013) Cemented, cementless, and hybrid prostheses for total hip replacement: a cost-effectiveness analysis. *BMJ*, vol 346, f1026.

Pritchard A (2004) Measuring government health services output in the UK national accounts: the new methodology and further analysis. *Economic Trends*, no 613, pp 69–81.

Szende A, Oppe M, Devlin N (eds) (2007) *EQ-5D Value Sets: Inventory, comparative review and user guide*. EuroQol Group monographs Volume 2. Dordrecht, The Netherlands: Springer.

CHAPTER 8

Where next for patient reported outcomes?

The importance and relevance of the patient's own views about their health is clear. The purpose of health care is to improve patient health and what constitutes an 'improvement' should obviously reflect what is important from the patient's perspective.

PRO questionnaires can provide a robust and reliable way of capturing the subjective views of patients. PROs have been around for decades and are already a central part of the evidence considered in health technology appraisal (HTA) systems around the world.

The 'state of the art' in developing, testing and analysing PRO data has, during this time, also been progressing – modern psychometric techniques provide ever better ways of ensuring that PROs are valid and reliable measures of patients' self-reported health.

Against that backdrop, the use of PROs by organisations such as Bupa, the English NHS and, increasingly, health systems around the world, represents a new and hugely innovative use of PROs: the *routine* collection of PRO data from patients as part of administrative data (in contrast to the use of PROs in clinical trials, observational studies or population surveys) is a new and notable development. The *use* of 'real world' PRO data to monitor and drive quality improvement at the health system level is, arguably, a critical break-through in health care management. It establishes a new benchmark in patient-centred health care delivery, with important implications for health systems internationally.

We have, in this book, highlighted the powerful ways that outcome data from patients can be used to inform patients' choices of treatments and providers; clinicians' shared decisions about treatment options and the purchasing decisions of budget holders in health care systems about what treatments to fund and from whom. PRO data can be used both by the providers of health care in internally managing their performance; and by commissioners and regulators or health care systems in externally auditing the quality of care. PRO data have the potential to be a real game-changer in the delivery of health care – a disruptive technology that requires all parties-patients, doctors, hospitals, budget-holders, regulators and policy makers-to sit up and pay attention to patients' views about health and health care.

That said, there is much work needed to realise the potential of PROs at the health system level.

Lessons and challenges

So, what might be learned from the experience of the English NHS PROMs programme? What are the key lessons for other health care systems and what challenges remain?

Using Patient Reported Outcomes to Improve Health Care,
First Edition. John Appleby, Nancy Devlin and David Parkin.
© 2016 John Wiley & Sons, Ltd. Published 2016 by John Wiley & Sons, Ltd.

The first conclusion to note from the English NHS PROMs programme (and indeed from Bupa's use of PROs that preceded it) is that it is possible to collect PRO data from patients as part of the routine delivery of care and also to obtain follow-up data from patients so that changes in health can be tracked. The logistical, ethical and other challenges in collecting data can be managed and the response rates that have been achieved are impressive.

Secondly, the data that are generated have been enthusiastically used to facilitate a wide range of analyses that, as we have shown in this book, can inform decisions by patients, clinicians, hospitals, health care budget holders and regulators.

Thirdly, a significant new expansion of the PROMs programme in England has been to extend the collection of data to the regular GP Patient Survey. Carried out quarterly and with responses from the public of around 900 000, the addition of the EQ-5D–5L to these surveys provide a valuable epidemiological insight into variations in health status across the country and by GP practice, as well as providing a potential to link to patient reported outcome data collected in hospitals.

Nevertheless, since the introduction of its PROMs programme in 2009, the English NHS has been slow to expand routine data collection beyond the initial four areas of elective surgery. And despite 5 years of data collection and analytical effort, the NHS is still struggling with how best to present the results to users in such a way that it can be readily understood and used by all stakeholders. The data are under used and many potential users poorly informed about the existence of PROMs information.

Despite patient choice being the initial catalyst to the introduction of PROs, the data have yet to be included in the patient choice website designed for patients choosing where to get their surgery. It is difficult to find specific examples of decisions that were informed by PRO data, or hard evidence on improvements in quality of care that have resulted from the data. Much of the potential of the data has yet to be realised.

The key lesson for other health care systems is that as much, if not *more*, effort needs to be devoted to how data can be presented and used by stakeholders, as to the logistics of data collection. Indeed, the introduction of PROs as part of routine data collection should ask, at every point along the way:
- Who will use these data?
- How will the data be used?
- How can we make sure the investment in these data generates value for the health care system?
- How can we make sure the data generates real improvements in quality of care?

A further challenge is how best to collect and analyse data in interventions other than elective surgery. The four surgical procedures that have been and continue to be the focus of the English NHS PROMs programme present relatively straightforward opportunities for measurement: surgery is planned and is a discrete event, which is delivered by a single provider. In contrast, treatment for many long term conditions comprises complex packages of health and social care, delivered by multiple providers, with variations in the nature, frequency and quality of care. There is no simple 'before and after' with these interventions, so the frequency with which patients should be asked to complete PROs requires careful consideration. Furthermore, the attribution of observed changes in health to the delivery of care and treatment being received by those patients presents a much more challenging task.

Finally, data collection and analysis in the English NHS has tended to take place in a top down way: data collection is mandated and the data collection system has a primary focus on getting the data back for centralised analysis and reporting. While this has been success-fully achieved, what is lost in this process is an opportunity for the data to be used by those to whom it most directly relevant: the patients who have completed the questionnaires, and their doctors, at the point treatment decisions are made. Notably, patients do not 'own' their own PRO data, and there is no process currently in place for them to see their own data. However, since 2012, patient level PROMs data can be made available (with the patient's consent) to individual clinicians for use in their clinical work.

The future development of PROMs could require a fundamentally different paradigm. Pa-tients could own their own PRO data: completing the PRO questionnaires online, enabling them to monitor their own health over time and to compare it with the health of others in the general population, of their own age, sex and other background characteristics and with others with similar conditions. PRO data can be shared with clinicians at appointments, and form the basis for conversations about health and treatment options. The data, in ano-nymised form, could be pooled and linked to administrative data sets, to serve the needs of other decision makers, such as providers, commissioners and regulators.

Not just as a nurse, but as a pioneering 'passionate statistician' (Magnello, 2010), there's no doubt that Florence Nightingale would be impressed with the expansion of her three health states – relieved, unrelieved and dead – to the 3125 possible health states[5] described by a questionnaire such as the EQ-5D-5L with five questions and five possible answers per question. She would also be impressed with examples, such as the English NHS, of the scale of the routine collection of patient reported outcomes. But as a nurse and tireless campaigner to improve the knowledge and use of health statistics, she would be the first to point out that the collection of patient reported outcome data is not an end in itself; its value lies in its use.

References

Magnello ME (2010) The passionate statistician. In: NelsonS, RaffertyAQM (eds.) *Notes on Nightingale: The Influence and Legacy of a Nursing Icon*. Cornell University Press, pp 114–129.

[5] For Florence Nightingale even data themselves apparently had a positive impact on her health state: 'Her enjoyment [of statistics] was so immense that she found that the sight of a long column of figures was "perfectly reviving".' (Magnello, 2010).

APPENDIX 1

PROM questionnaire that is currently completed by patients after undergoing varicose vein surgery. (Reproduced with permission of Health and Social Care Information Centre.)

NHS

Varicose Veins Surgery Questionnaire

After your operation

About three months ago you had a Varicose Veins Operation. You may remember that you agreed that we could send you an *After your operation* questionnaire. Please can you fill in this questionnaire and return it using the provided pre-paid envelope. Thank you for your help.

Q1. Is anyone helping you fill in this questionnaire?

Yes ☐₁   No ☐₂

If the answer is yes, please give the relationship to you of the person assisting you

[ ]

Q2. What is your date of birth?

[D][D] [M][M] [1][9][Y][Y]

A question about your current home circumstances

Q3. Which statement best describes your living arrangements?

I live with partner/spouse/family/friends ☐₁

I live alone ☐₂

I live in a nursing home, hospital or other long-term care home ☐₃

Other ☐₄

Q4. Please confirm when your varicose veins operation took place (day, month, year).

[D][D] [M][M] [2][0][Y][Y]

1

Using Patient Reported Outcomes to Improve Health Care,
First Edition. John Appleby, Nancy Devlin and David Parkin.
© 2016 John Wiley & Sons, Ltd. Published 2016 by John Wiley & Sons, Ltd.

Appendix 1

Varicose Veins Surgery Questionnaire – After your operation

Some questions about your surgery and your health
Please mark the boxes below with a tick or numbers where appropriate.
If you are unsure about how to answer a question, please give the best
answer you can.

**Q5. Did you experience any of the following problems after your
operation? Please tick *Yes* or *No* for each problem.**

	Yes	No
Allergy or reaction to drug	☐₁	☐₂
Urinary problems	☐₁	☐₂
Bleeding	☐₁	☐₂
Wound problems	☐₁	☐₂

**Q6. Have you been readmitted to hospital since the operation
on your varicose veins?**

Yes ☐₁   No ☐₂

Q7. Have you had another operation on your varicose veins?

Yes ☐₁   No ☐₂

Q8. In general, would you say your health is:

Excellent ☐₁   Very good ☐₂   Good ☐₃   Fair ☐₄   Poor ☐₅

Q9. How would you describe the results of your operation?

Excellent ☐₁   Very good ☐₂   Good ☐₃   Fair ☐₄   Poor ☐₅

SAMPLE

Varicose Veins Surgery Questionnaire – After your operation

Q10. Overall, how are the problems now with your varicose veins on which you had surgery, compared to before your operation?

Much better	A little better	About the same	A little worse	Much worse
☐₁	☐₂	☐₃	☐₄	☐₅

The following questions relate to problems commonly associated with varicose veins. We appreciate that you may no longer have any visible varicose veins after your surgery but please try and answer each question as best you can.

Q11. Do you have any visible varicose veins on your legs at the moment?
(*Please tick one box for each leg*)

	Right Leg	Left Leg
Yes	☐₁	☐₂
No	☐₁	☐₂

Q12. If Yes, please draw in your visible varicose veins in the diagram(s) below. If No, please proceed to Q13.

Legs viewed from front   Legs viewed from back

Varicose Veins Surgery Questionnaire – After your operation

Q13. In the last two weeks, for how many days did your varicose veins cause you pain or ache?
(Please tick one box for each leg)

	Right Leg	Left Leg
None at all	☐₁	☐₂
Between 1 and 5 days	☐₁	☐₂
Between 6 and 10 days	☐₁	☐₂
For more than 10 days	☐₁	☐₂

Q14. During the last two weeks, on how many days did you take painkilling tablets for your varicose veins?
(Please tick one box)

None at all	☐₁
Between 1 and 5 days	☐₂
Between 6 and 10 days	☐₃
For more than 10 days	☐₄

Q15. In the last two weeks, how much ankle swelling have you had?
(Please tick one box)

None at all	☐₁
Severe ankle swelling	☐₂
Moderate ankle swelling (e.g. causing you to sit with your feet up wherever possible)	☐₃
Severe ankle swelling (e.g. causing you difficulty putting on your shoes)	☐₄

Q16. In the last two weeks, have you worn support tights or stockings?
(Please tick one box for each leg)

	Right Leg	Left Leg
No	☐₁	☐₂
Yes, those I bought myself without a doctor's prescription	☐₁	☐₂
Yes, those my doctor prescribed for me which I wear occasionally	☐₁	☐₂
Yes, those my doctor prescribed for me which I wear every day	☐₁	☐₂

Q17. In the last two weeks, have you had any itching in association with your varicose veins?
(Please tick one box for each leg)

	Right Leg	Left Leg
No	☐₁	☐₂
Yes, but only above the knee	☐₁	☐₂
Yes, but only below the knee	☐₁	☐₂
Both above and below the knee	☐₁	☐₂

Q18. Do you have purple discolouration caused by tiny blood vessels in the skin, in association with your varicose veins?
(Please tick one box for each leg)

	Right Leg	Left Leg
Yes	☐₁	☐₂
No	☐₁	☐₂

Appendix 1

Varicose Veins Surgery Questionnaire – After your operation

Q19. Do you have any rash or eczema in the area of your ankle?
(Please tick one box for each leg)

	Right Leg	Left Leg
No	☐₁	☐₂
Yes, but it does not require any treatment from a doctor or district nurse	☐₁	☐₂
Yes, and it requires treatment from my doctor or district nurse	☐₁	☐₂

Q20. Do you have a skin ulcer associated with your varicose veins?
(Please tick one box for each leg)

	Right Leg	Left Leg
Yes	☐₁	☐₂
No	☐₁	☐₂

Q21. Does the appearance of your varicose veins cause you concern?
(Please tick one box for each leg)

	Right Leg	Left Leg
No	☐₁	☐₂
Their appearance causes me slight concern	☐₁	☐₂
Yes, their appearance causes me a great deal of concern	☐₁	☐₂

Q22. Does the appearance of your varicose veins influence your choice of clothing including tights?
(Please tick one box)

No	☐₁
Occasionally	☐₂
Often	☐₃
Always	☐₄

SAMPLE

Varicose Veins Surgery Questionnaire – After your operation

Q23. During the last two weeks, have your varicose veins interfered with your work/housework or other daily activities?
(Please tick one box)

No ☐₁

I have been able to work but my work has suffered to some extent ☐₂

I have been able to work but my work has suffered to a moderate extent ☐₃

My veins have prevented me from working one day or more ☐₄

Q24. During the last two weeks, have your varicose veins interfered with your leisure activities (including sport, hobbies and social life)?
(Please tick one box)

No ☐₁

Yes, my enjoyment has suffered to a slight extent ☐₂

Yes, my enjoyment has suffered to a moderate extent ☐₃

My veins have prevented me from taking part in any leisure activities ☐₄

Varicose Veins Surgery Questionnaire – After your operation

By placing a tick in one box in each group (Questions 25–29) below, please indicate which statements best describe your own health state today.

Q25. Mobility

I have no problems in walking about ☐1

I have some problems in walking about ☐2

I am confined to bed ☐3

Q26. Self-Care

I have no problems with self-care ☐1

I have some problems washing or dressing myself ☐2

I am unable to wash or dress myself ☐3

Q27. Usual Activities
(*e.g. work, study, housework, family or leisure activities*)

I have no problems with performing my usual activities ☐1

I have some problems with performing my usual activities ☐2

I am unable to perform my usual activities ☐3

Q28. Pain/Discomfort

I have no pain or discomfort ☐1

I have moderate pain or discomfort ☐2

I have extreme pain or discomfort ☐3

Q29. Anxiety/Depression

I am not anxious or depressed ☐1

I am moderately anxious or depressed ☐2

I am extremely anxious or depressed ☐3

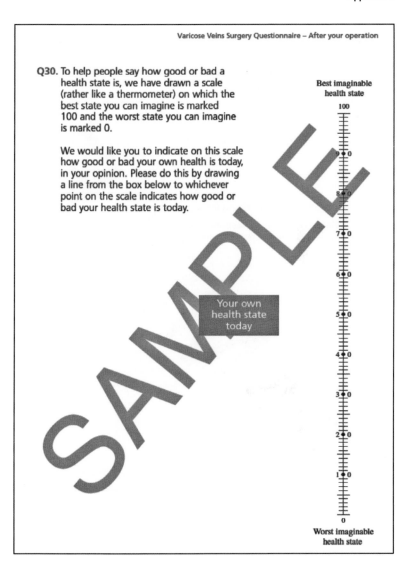

Q30. To help people say how good or bad a health state is, we have drawn a scale (rather like a thermometer) on which the best state you can imagine is marked 100 and the worst state you can imagine is marked 0.

We would like you to indicate on this scale how good or bad your own health is today, in your opinion. Please do this by drawing a line from the box below to whichever point on the scale indicates how good or bad your health state is today.

Your own health state today

Best imaginable health state

100

90

80

70

60

50

40

30

20

10

0

Worst imaginable health state

Varicose Veins Surgery Questionnaire – After your operation

Q31. Today's date (day, month, year)

| D | D | | M | M | | 2 | 0 | Y | Y |

Q32. Do you consider yourself to have a disability?

Yes   No

☐₁   ☐₂

Thank you for your assistance.

**Please return this questionnaire in the envelope provided.
You do not have to use a stamp – the postage is already paid.**

SAMPLE

APPENDIX 2

The EQ-5D-5L©. (Reproduced with permission of EuroQol Group. © 2009 EuroQol Group. EQ-5D™ is a trademark of the EuroQol Group.)

By placing a tick in one box in each group below, please indicate which statements best describe your own health state TODAY.

MOBILITY

I have no problems in walking about ☐
I have slight problems in walking about ☐
I have moderate problems in walking about ☐
I have severe problems in walking about ☐
I am unable to walk about ☐

SELF-CARE

I have no problems washing or dressing myself ☐
I have slight problems washing or dressing myself ☐
I have moderate problems washing or dressing myself ☐
I have severe problems washing or dressing myself ☐
I am unable to wash or dress myself ☐

USUAL ACTIVITIES *(e.g. work, study, housework, family or leisure activities)*

I have no problems doing my usual activities ☐
I have slight problems doing my usual activities ☐
I have moderate problems doing my usual activities ☐
I have severe problems doing my usual activities ☐
I am unable to do my usual activities ☐

PAIN / DISCOMFORT

I have no pain or discomfort ☐
I have slight pain or discomfort ☐
I have moderate pain or discomfort ☐
I have severe pain or discomfort ☐
I have extreme pain or discomfort ☐

ANXIETY / DEPRESSION

I am not anxious or depressed ☐
I am slightly anxious or depressed ☐
I am moderately anxious or depressed ☐
I am severely anxious or depressed ☐
I am extremely anxious or depressed ☐

Using Patient Reported Outcomes to Improve Health Care,
First Edition. John Appleby, Nancy Devlin and David Parkin.
© 2016 John Wiley & Sons, Ltd. Published 2016 by John Wiley & Sons, Ltd.

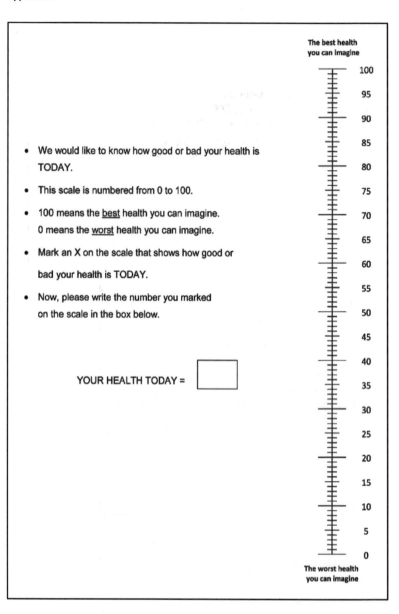

The best health you can imagine

- We would like to know how good or bad your health is TODAY.

- This scale is numbered from 0 to 100.

- 100 means the <u>best</u> health you can imagine.
  0 means the <u>worst</u> health you can imagine.

- Mark an X on the scale that shows how good or bad your health is TODAY.

- Now, please write the number you marked on the scale in the box below.

YOUR HEALTH TODAY =

The worst health you can imagine

100
95
90
85
80
75
70
65
60
55
50
45
40
35
30
25
20
15
10
5
0

Dr Tim Hughes' shared decision-making aid for patients. (Reproduced with permission of Tim Hughes.)

Helping patients decide what to do

One way to help you decide what to do when you are faced with a decision about an operation is called **Shared Decision Making**. It's all about us giving you all the information you need about your options, exploring your preferences and values with you and then helping you use all of this to make a decision about the right treatment for you.Our COD here is about understanding your **C**hoice and **O**ptions and making a good **D**ecision for you.

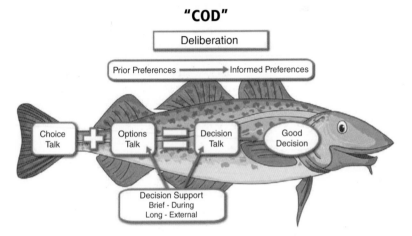

There are a number of Shared Decision Making tools that can help you understand more about your Choice and Options before making a Decision that might affect the rest of your life.

Visit www.valeofyorkccg.nhs.uk and click on the Shared Decision Making picture.

There are some more on the Patient.co.uk website, one of the best websites for information for patients: www.patient.co.uk/decision-aids

Patient reported outcome measures: PROMS

One useful piece of information for you is knowing what other patients who have had your operation thought about having it done, after they had had that operation. This information is called PROMS, Patient Reported Outcome Measures. PROMs are obtained

Using Patient Reported Outcomes to Improve Health Care,
First Edition. John Appleby, Nancy Devlin and David Parkin.
© 2016 John Wiley & Sons, Ltd. Published 2016 by John Wiley & Sons, Ltd.

by getting patients who have previously had certain problems complete questionnaires on their symptoms, condition and overall quality of life both before and after their surgery. Different questionnaires give us different scores and information about different conditions and operations. Some can be used for any condition, such as the EQ-5D for health-related quality of life and some are only useful for specific conditions, such as the Oxford Hip and Knee Score and Aberdeen Varicose Vein Score.

Different types of PROMs questionnaires.

EQ-5D index score	• Multi-dimensional – five areas
	  1. mobility
	  2. self-care
	  3. usual activities
	  4. pain/discomfort
	  5. anxiety/depression
	• Responses record three levels of severity
	• Scores are weighted and combined to give a single index

EQ-5D Visual Analogue Scale (VAS)	• Self rating health related quality of life • Places self reported health state on a point in a line • Line ranges from 0 to 100 where 0 is worst and 100 best possible health
Oxford **Hip** Score	• Specific for Total Hip Replacements • 12 questions to assess function and pain, 0–4 points • Given as a single summed score from 0 to 48 • national average scores(2012) pre-op = 18.07 post-op = 38.35
Oxford **Knee** Score	• Specific for Total Knee Replacements • 12 questions to assess function and pain, 0–4 points • Given as a single summed score from 0 to 48
Aberdeen **Varicose Vein** Questionnaire	• Specific for Varicose Veins. • Questions on amount of pain experienced; ankle swelling; use of support stockings; interference with social and domestic activities and the cosmetic aspects of varicose veins. • The score is a value from 0 to 100, where 0 is 'best' and 100 is 'worst'.

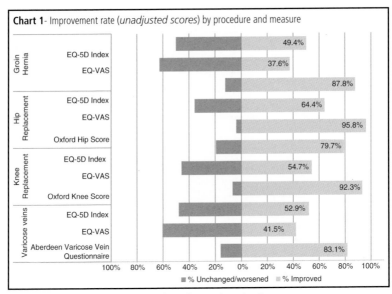

Chart 1- Improvement rate (*unadjusted scores*) by procedure and measure

Reproduced with permission of Health and Social Care Information Centre.

Index

Using Patient Reported Outcomes to Improve Health Care,
First Edition. John Appleby, Nancy Devlin and David Parkin.
© 2016 John Wiley & Sons, Ltd. Published 2016 by John Wiley & Sons, Ltd.